Gas Monitoring and Pulse Oximetry

J.S. Gravenstein, M.D., Dr.h.c.

Graduate Research Professor
Department of Anesthesiology
University of Florida College of Medicine
Gainesville, Florida

Butterworth–Heinemann
Boston London Singapore Sydney Toronto Wellington

Every effort has been made to ensure that the drug dosage schedules within this text are accurate and conform to standards accepted at time of publication. However, as treatment recommendations vary in the light of continuing research and clinical experience, the reader is advised to verify drug dosage schedules herein with information found on product information sheets. This is especially true in cases of new or infrequently used drugs.

Recognizing the importance of preserving what has been written, it is the policy of Butterworth–Heinemann to have the books it publishes and we exert our best efforts to that end.

Library of Congress Cataloging-in-Publication Data

Gravenstein, J.S.
Gas monitoring and pulse oximetry /Joachim S. Gravenstein.
p. cm.
Includes bibliographical references.
ISBN 0-409-90261-6
1. Anesthesiology. 2. Oximetry. 3. Patient monitoring.
4. Modell, Jerome H., 1932– . I. Modell, Jerome H., 1932– .
II. Title.
[DNLM: 1. Anesthesia. 2. Monitoring, Physiology.
3. Oximetry.
WO 200 G776g]
RD82.G724 1990
617.9'6—dc20
DNLM/DLC
for Library of Congress 90–1328

British Library Cataloguing in Publication Data

Gravenstein, Joachim S. (Joachim S. Joachim Stefan) 1925–
Gas monitoring and pulse oximetry.
1. Medicine. Anaesthesia. Monitoring
I. Title
617.96

ISBN 0-409-90261-6

Butterworth–Heinemann
80 Montvale Avenue
Stoneham, MA 02180

10 9 8 7 6 5 4 3 2 1

Printed in the United States of America

Dedicated on August 5, 1989,
to Jerome H. Modell, M.D.,
for twenty years the exemplary chairman of
the Department of Anesthesiology,
University of Florida

Contents

Preface

A substantial part of the practice of anesthesia is devoted to ventilation of the patient's lungs and to the administration of oxygen and inhalation anesthetics (Figure i), during which many questions about anesthetic administration and ventilation are raised in the mind of the clinician (Figure ii). This book addresses these questions and offers brief answers.

In the introduction, justification for monitoring gases and oxygenation is presented. Next comes a primer on clinical gas monitoring and pulse oximetry. The remainder of the book comprises an outline of concepts underlying the uptake and distribution of anesthetics, anesthesia breathing systems, ventilation and perfusion, and the relevant technology of monitoring.

The book is kept brief because it was written for the busy clinician. For physiologic, physical, or engineering details, the reader is referred to more exhaustive treatises listed in the references.

J.S.G.

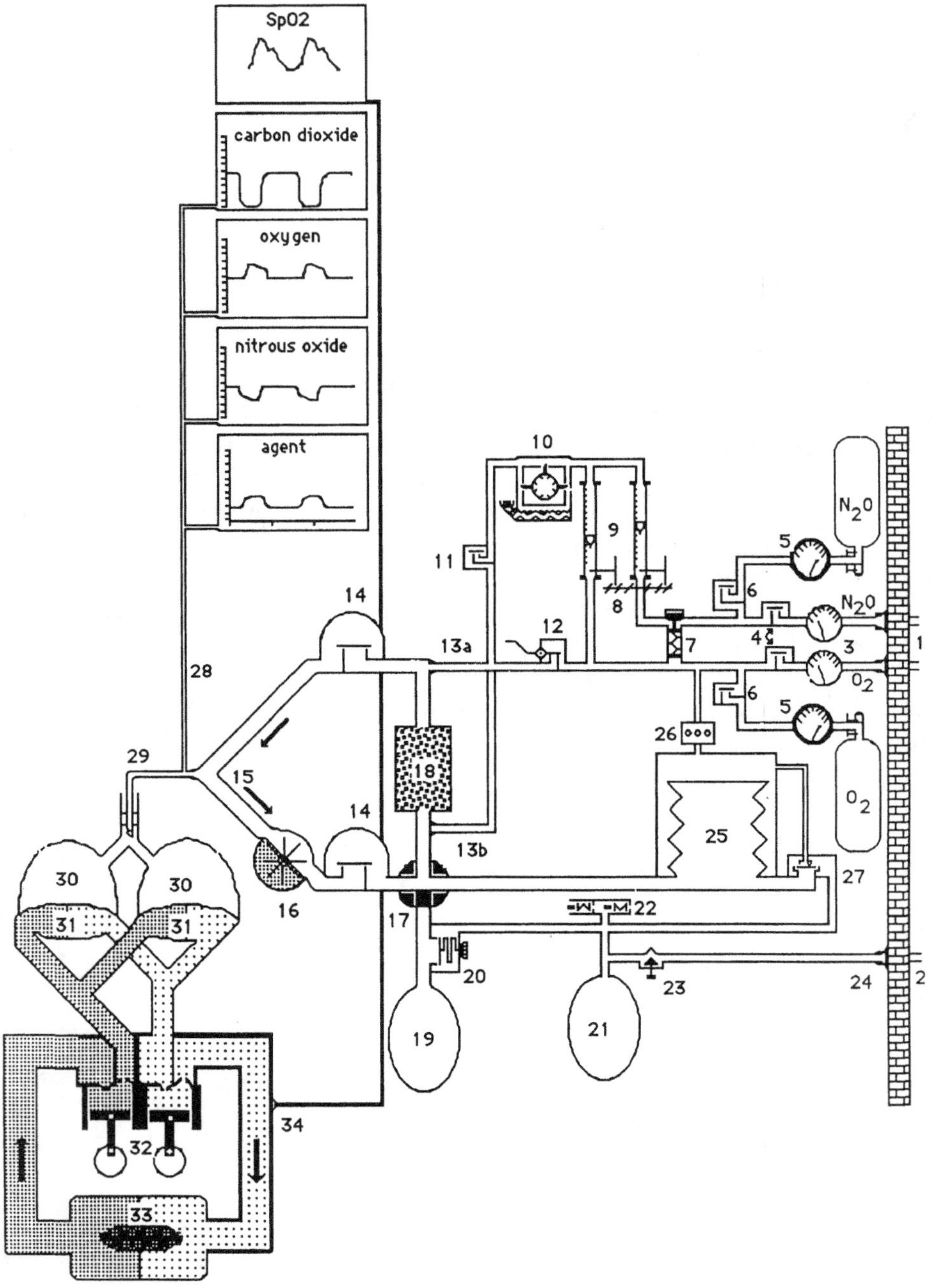

FIGURE i *Generic anesthesia machine. The features of this machine are shown with easy-to-understand symbols rather than with engineering icons. The symbols represent function rather than design. SpO_2 denotes saturation of hemoglobin with oxygen, as estimated by pulse oximetry.*

Gas Supply

1. Central gas supply
2. Central vacuum

3. Pressure gauges for piped oxygen and nitrous oxide
4. One-way valve: prevents loss of gas when hoses carrying piped gases are disconnected
5. Pressure gauges for oxygen and nitrous oxide cylinders, with pressure-regulating function
6. Valves preventing flow of oxygen (nitrous oxide) from cylinders, as long as pipes carrying gas from the central gas supply are connected and pressurized
7. Oxygen-pressure failure protection ("oxygen fail-safe"): stops nitrous oxide flow when oxygen pressure falls
8. Oxygen proportioning device: makes it impossible to deliver less than preset proportion of oxygen (usually 25%) in gas mixture
9. Flowmeter tubes and floats
10. Vaporizer
11. Device that minimizes pressure transmission from breathing circuit to vaporizer
12. Oxygen flush valve
13. Common gas outlets, (a) between inspiratory valve and absorber, and (b) between absorber and expiratory valve

Breathing Circuit

14. Inspiratory and expiratory valves
15. Y piece
16. Bidirectional respirometer
17. Selector switch
18. Carbon dioxide absorber
19. Breathing bag
20. Adjustable pressure-limiting (APL), or "pop-off," valve
21. Scavenging reservoir bag
22. Valve to compensate for excessive pressure or excessive suction
23. Control for adjusting suction
24. Connection to central vacuum

Ventilator

25. Ventilator bellows
26. Ventilator power supply (here, oxygen) and controls
27. Ventilator pressure-relief valve: dumps gas from breathing circuit to scavenging system late in expiration, when bellows reaches top of box

Gas Monitoring System

28. Capillary, through which gas is aspirated for analysis

Physiologic System

29. Endotracheal tube
30. Lungs
31. Pulmonary capillary bed
32. Heart, with atria and ventricles
33. Peripheral capillary beds

Pulse Oximetry

34. Pulse oximeter probe attached to detect arterial pulsation

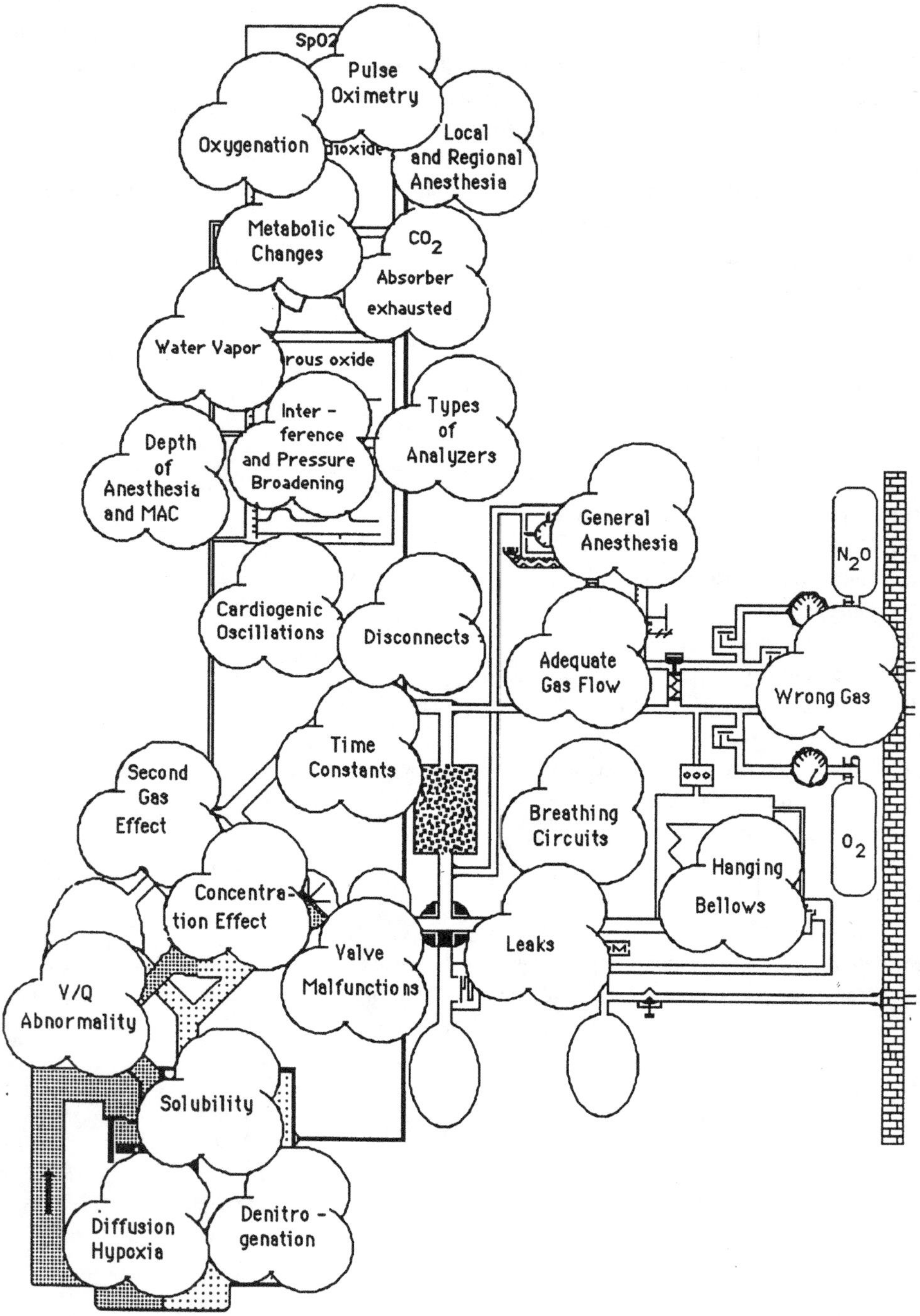

FIGURE ii *Questions about anesthesia. The clouds represent questions that arise in the clinician's mind concerning the functions of the anesthesia machine and circle breathing system (Figure i) and the patient. MAC denotes minimum alveolar concentration; V/Q, ventilation-to-perfusion ratio.*

Acknowledgments

This little book was skillfully edited by Ingrid Mellone and Lynn Dirk and patiently reviewed for conceptual mistakes by Drs. J. van der Aa, M.L. Good, N. Gravenstein, S. Lampotang, D.A. Paulus, and K. Mollgaard, who first suggested the need for this modest monograph.

Chapter 1

Introduction

The first monitors in anesthesia were eyes glued on the patient, a finger on the pulse, and ears cocked to hear breath and heart sounds. These are still the most important monitors. Their application requires practice, skill, and one instrument: the stethoscope. The good clinician will not proceed without them.

Several electronic monitoring devices have joined inspection, palpation, and auscultation during anesthesia in the operating room and wherever anesthetists work. The clinician can monitor critical variables that cannot be perceived by the unaided human senses, such as the concentrations of oxygen and carbon dioxide in respired gas, with electronic monitors. They also help quantify variables that the human eye, hand, or ear can assess only qualitatively. These monitors help watch patient, machine, breathing circuit, and ventilator. Electronic monitors do not tire, can repeat measurements with monotonous regularity, and do so without encouragement (other than electricity). Such monitors include the manometer (airway, noninvasive blood pressure), electrocardiograph (ECG), nerve stimulator, devices to measure gas flow and concentration, thermometer, pulse oximeter, electroencephalograph (EEG), and invasive probes to measure intravascular pressures and concentrations of gases or ions.

Every patient is monitored with noninvasive instruments, although some also require invasive monitoring. Reliance on the traditional noninvasive devices—namely, the sphygmomanometer (automatic or manual) and the electrocardiogram (ECG)—is so universal in modern anesthesia practice that monitoring blood pressure (BP) and obtaining an ECG have become requisite even in minor procedures. Clinicians believe that a certain degree of hypotension—or, about as often, hypertension (as reported by the sphygmomanometer)—requires attention and correction.[1-4] The timely detection of cardiac arrest, an ischemic change of the ST segment, or a malignant arrhythmia justifies the ECG. No wonder that the sphygmomanometer and electrocardiograph have been labeled essential monitors in clinical practice; no practitioner would want to do without them.

Don't be fooled, though. Essential monitors leave wide gaps because they fail to identify many important and potentially serious problems. Trouble may be brewing in a patient under general anesthesia with no change in BP and no evidence of distress in the ECG (Table 1.1). Indeed, hypoxemia may have already damaged the brain, even if neither arterial pressure values nor ECG give any hint of this disaster. Cheney

Table 1.1 Comparison of Monitors in Terms of Timely Indication of Trouble

	Cardiac Arrest	*Shock*	*Hyperpyrexia*	*Low Fraction of Inspired Oxygen*	*Machine Error*	*Depth of Anesthesia*
Sphygmomanometer	Yes	Yes	No*	No*	No	Yes†
Electrocardiograph	Yes	No‡	No*	No*	No	No
Thermometer	No	No	Yes	No	No	No
Pulse oximeter	Yes	Yes§	No	Yes¶	Yes‖	No
Capnograph	Yes**	Yes**	Yes	No	Yes	No**
Oxygraph††	Yes**	Yes**	Yes‡‡	Yes	Yes§§	No**
Anesthetigraph¶¶	Yes‖‖	Yes‖‖	No	No	Yes***	Yes

The table assumes a rapidly responding oxygen analyzer (oxygraph) that permits the determination of inspired and expired oxygen concentration. Machine errors include disconnections, leaks, valve malfunctions, and wrong gas connections.

* Nonspecific changes until severe hyperpyrexia or hypoxemia have affected the heart and brain.
† BP changes are often used as a guide in adjusting depth of anesthesia; BP is an indirect indicator of depth of anesthesia.
‡ The ECG will show changes when shock lasts long enough or is severe enough.
§ The pulse oximeter may fail to function in shock.
¶ The pulse oximeter will show the consequences of an unphysiologically low fraction of inspired oxygen ($F_{I}O_2$), but not as early as will the oxygen analyzer in the breathing circuit.
‖ If machine malfunction leads to hypoxemia.
** The capnograph and oxygraph reflect decreasing cardiac output (after arrest, during shock, or with deep anesthesia), which causes less oxygen to be taken up by the lungs and less carbon dioxide to be delivered to them.
†† Monitor of oxygen in respired gas.
‡‡ Increased oxygen consumption is expected.
§§ If malfunction leads to low fraction of inspired oxygen.
¶¶ Monitor of anesthetic agents in respired gas.
‖‖ With low or no pulmonary blood flow, uptake of inhalation anesthetics is expected to be affected.
*** If machine error affects anesthetic concentration in respired gas.

examined hundreds of anesthesia records that had found their way into the hands of malpractice insurance carriers because the patients in question had suffered harm during anesthesia.[5] He concluded that difficulty with ventilation was by far the most common cause of disaster. Yet these mishaps occurred when arterial pressure monitors and ECGs were already established as almost universal monitors during anesthesia. Tinker et al. estimated that capnography and pulse oximetry could have proven helpful in the prevention of serious mishaps in anesthesia: capnography in 2% of patients under general anesthesia and 1% of patients under regional anesthesia, pulse oximetry in 40% of patients under general anesthesia and 80% of patients under regional anesthesia. The combination of capnography and pulse oximetry, in the words of the authors, was "considered potentially preventative in 93% of preventable mishaps."[6]

Some national societies are now encouraging or mandating the use of pulse oximetry and capnography.[7,8] In addition to the sphygmomanometer and ECG, therefore, a second tier of monitors arises. This includes the pulse oximeter and analyzers of gases entering and leaving the patient's airway. These monitors have been called simple, safe, and cost-effective.[9] Since the monitors measure only the concentration of inspired and expired gases and the saturation of hemoglobin in arterial blood, one would at first assume that the information derived from them would generate intelligence on matters relating to ventilation only. This is not true. They generate much information on circulation and metabolism (Table 1.1). In contrast, the traditional essential monitors (sphygmomanometer and ECG) can reveal changes in the cardiovascular system, but when respired gases are dangerously abnormal or when ventilation lags, these first-tier monitors are silent until the patient is severely affected.

The value of gas monitors and pulse oximeters has been challenged. Sykes, for example, worries that the profusion of monitors leads to an "abrogation of personal contact with the patient and reliance on monitors—[which] is a recipe for disaster."[10] Orkin accumulated statistics to show that the decline in anesthetic mortality preceded the widespread use of capnography and pulse oximetry.[11] He wonders whether the application of expensive monitors can be justified when so little additional benefit is gained. Indeed, he worries about possible harm arising from the employment of more and more mechanical and electronic devices. They might distract, mislead, or lull the clinician into inattention. These serious concerns deserve consideration. They focus our attention on the purpose of our entire effort—namely, to make anesthesia safe and to do so at the lowest possible cost.

First, a word about cost. Monitoring accounts for a small fraction of the expenses of surgery (including surgeon's fees and operating room costs), hospitalization, and all the attendant examinations and drugs; not to be forgotten is the loss of income suffered by the patient. We estimate that comprehensive noninvasive monitoring, consisting of automated sphygmomanometry, electrocardiography, respired gas monitoring, and pulse oximetry, costs between $10 and $20 per patient,[12] whereas effects and treatment of the disease will consume many thousands of dollars per patient.

Operating time is expensive. If gas monitoring would make it possible to shorten the patient's time of recovery from anesthesia and thus the time between the end of operation and the moment the responsive patient can leave the operating room, the gas monitor would soon pay for itself: a minute of operating room time costs about $10.00, but gas monitoring during an entire anesthetic costs only about $2.50 per patient.[13] We spend less than 1% of the total cost of a surgically treated disease on safety—usually far less than 1%. That is a bargain when we remember that more preventable disasters occur during anesthesia and recovery from anesthesia than during any other time of a patient's stay in the hospital.[14]

How much safety do we buy for this small sum of $2.50 per patient? We could measure safety scientifically by assessing the outcome of anesthesia. How did the patient fare during and after the operation? Here we must deal with two factors and then look for a relationship between them. First, we must ask whether the patient's condition after the operation and anesthetic is worse than it was before. If the answer is yes, we must establish whether the anesthesia caused the deterioration. Did the patient's vital signs veer beyond limits considered safe? Did the oxygen saturation fall dangerously low?

The demonstration of causal relationships requires properly controlled prospective studies of large numbers of patients. Such studies, however, are nonexistent. The best we have is the experience of the insurance industry, which suggests that monitoring with the aim of early detection and prevention of hypoxia may help.[14] Other studies offer glimpses at trends rather than hard scientific evidence.[15]

Today we accept that monitoring arterial pressure and ECG is requisite for safe anesthesia. But even for these generally accepted monitoring methods, controlled outcome studies are not available.[16] Years ago we adopted sphygmomanometry and ECG for routine monitoring because thousands of anesthetists agreed that doing so was sensible. After all, when a patient's condition deteriorates, BP falls and the ECG changes. We never examined whether noticing the onset of these changes gave us enough warning to avert at least some of the disasters, although we generally accepted the assumption that early warnings were indeed helpful. Now we must ask ourselves whether we can trust our clinical judgment about the value of capnography and pulse oximetry, the two variables of advanced noninvasive monitoring most often discussed by doubters and proponents alike. Should we reject the clinical judgment of those who remind us that respiratory complications are more likely to kill our patients than cardiovascular or other complications? Should we mistrust our instinct that measuring oxygen and carbon dioxide in respired gas will give us early information on the status of oxygenation and ventilation? Should we limit ourselves to watching the patient for subjective evidence of cyanosis?[17] Or should we grasp the opportunity to discover, with the help of pulse oximetry, the earliest objective evidence of desaturation? Is the admittedly scientifically weak clinical evidence in favor of routine monitoring of BP and ECGs stronger than the rationale for adopting pulse oximetry and gas monitoring? I think not.

Outcome studies would answer the question—or would they? What endpoint should we look for? Clearly, death and devastating brain damage are unacceptable outcomes.[18,19] So are myocardial infarction and other permanent injuries that are often attributed to anesthesia and that could be prevented. But should we worry about transient problems such as arrhythmias or pulmonary congestion? If such complications do not prolong hospitalization or increase the cost of treatment, and if they are not harbingers of premature death, can they be shrugged off? I believe so, provided they do not affect the quality of life. And herein lies the crux of outcome studies.

We should not limit ourselves to a count of deaths from hypoxic devastation or myocardial infarction. Instead, we should insist on measurement of more subtle hypoxic damage. I am convinced that the effects of hypoxia do not follow an all-or-nothing law ("Either hypoxia kills the brain or does no harm at all"). Rather, there must be a spectrum of damage that ranges from death or devastation of the brain on one extreme to damage with barely perceptible neurologic or psychological deficits on the other. As with any extreme, the frequency of fatal hypoxia is likely to be lower than the frequency of severe to mild hypoxia. We have no data on how often mild hypoxia has caused patients to suffer some impairment, perhaps robbing them of their peak intellectual capacity without ruining their ability to maintain a job and function in the family. If this spectrum of damage exists, it is our responsibility to take all sensible steps to assure the patient of excellent ventilation and oxygenation at all times.

Toward this end, we are obliged to employ accepted anesthetic techniques, pay constant attention, and exploit all the assistance we can get from instruments that can discover abnormalities earlier and more reliably than the human senses. Should future outcome studies show that without support from such instruments, the best and the weakest among us are able to maintain good anesthetic technique at all times, sustain vigilance without fail, and exhibit quick responses even when fatigued or distracted, we can then put gas analyzers and pulse oximeters into a museum as evidence of well-intended but unnecessary precautions. Until that day, I would ask the anesthetist who cares for a member of my family or for me to please make use of the available tools, including gas monitoring and pulse oximetry.

REFERENCES

1. Amaranath L, Burke P, Kreul J, Kirilcuk V, Gravenstein JS: Why monitor? In: Gravenstein JS, Newbower RS, Ream AK, Smith N Ty, eds. Monitoring surgical patients in the operating room. Springfield, IL: CC Thomas, 1979:19–27
2. Steen PA, Tinker JH, Tarhan S: Myocardial reinfarction after anesthesia and surgery. JAMA 1978; 239:2566–2570
3. Eerola M, Eerola R, Kaukinen S, Kaukinen L: Risk factors in surgical patients with verified preoperative myocardial infarction. Acta Anaesth Scand 1980; 24:219–223
4. Goldman L, Caldera DL: Risks of general anesthesia and elective operation in the hypertensive patient. Anesthesiology 1979; 50:285–292
5. Cheney FW: Anesthesia: Potential risks and causes of incidents. In: Gravenstein JS, Holzer J, eds. Safety and cost containment in anesthesia. Stoneham, MA: Butterworths, 1988: 11–20
6. Tinker JH, Dull DL, Caplan RA, et al: Role of monitoring devices in prevention of anesthetic mishaps: A closed claims analysis. Anesthesiology 1989; 71:541–546
7. American Society of Anesthesiologists Standards for Basic Intra-operative Monitoring (Approved October 21, 1986): Newsletter of the Anesthesia Patient Safety Foundation, Park Ridge, IL, March 1987, p 3
8. Faculty of Anaesthetists RACS: Policy Statement, June 1988. Reprinted in the Newsletter of the Anesthesia Patient Safety Foundation, Park Ridge, IL, September 1988, p 23
9. Severinghaus JW: Continuous monitoring of alveolar and inspiratory concentrations of anesthetic and respiratory gases is safe, simple, and cost-effective. J Clin Monit 1987; 3:123

10. Sykes MK: Continuous monitoring of alveolar and inspiratory concentrations of anesthetic and respiratory gases is difficult and potentially unsafe. J Clin Monit 1987; 3:116–122
11. Orkin FK: Practice standards: The Midas touch or the emperor's new clothes? Anesthesiology 1989; 70:567–571
12. Gravenstein JS, Paulus DA, Montoya R: The cost of clinical monitoring. In, Aldrete JA, ed. The cost of anesthesia. New York: Springer Verlag, in press
13. Frazier WT: Strategies for gas monitoring. II. Integration (Multigas parameters). J Clin Monit 1987; 3:300–301
14. Wood M: Monitoring equipment and loss reduction: An insurer's view. In: Gravenstein JS, Holzer JF, eds. Safety and cost containment. Stoneham, MA: Butterworths, 1988: 47–54
15. Eichhorn JH: Prevention of intraoperative anesthesia accidents and related severe injury through safety monitoring. Anesthesiology 1989; 70:572–577
16. Gravenstein JS: Essential monitoring examined through different lenses. J Clin Monit 1986; 2:22–29
17. Comroe JH, Botelho S: The unreliability of cyanosis in the recognition of arterial anoxemia. Am J Med Sci 1947; 214:1
18. Brown DL: Anesthesia risk: A historical perspective. In: Brown DL, ed. Risk and outcome in anesthesia. Philadelphia: Lippincott; 1988
19. Ward RW, Lane MJ: Anesthesiology and medicolegal outcome. In: Brown DL, ed. Risk and outcome in anesthesia. Philadelphia: Lippincott; 1988

Chapter 2

Primer for Gas Monitoring and Pulse Oximetry

CAPNOGRAPHY

Monitoring carbon dioxide in inspired and end-tidal gas has set the standard for gas monitoring. The typical capnogram looks like the silhouette of a snake that has eaten an elephant (Figure 2.1). Usually there is no carbon dioxide in inspired gas, and the flat inspiratory phase of a capnogram merges with the baseline. This is called phase I (Figure 2.2). Then the capnogram takes off. In a fraction of a second the baseline rises steeply (up the posterior of the elephant). This is phase II of the capnogram, during which alveolar gas from the patient's lungs reaches the site where the analyzer either samples the gas for analysis (sidestream) or measures the concentration of carbon dioxide directly (mainstream). During the respiratory pause, gas containing carbon dioxide continues to fill the tube that carries the patient's respired gas (Figure 2.3). The carbon dioxide remains there until the next breath is drawn by the patient or pushed into his or her lungs by the ventilator. As long as the gas sits waiting for the next inspiration, the capnogram inscribes a plateau (the flat back of the elephant); this is phase III. The next breath then arrives and sweeps away the carbon dioxide. The capnogram rapidly tumbles back to zero (down the front of the elephant). This descending part of the capnogram is phase IV. Many sophisticated analyses of capnography have been published, and alternative methods of presenting carbon dioxide data have been proposed.[1]

The capnogram sets the rhythm for gas monitoring. The waveform shows when inspiration starts and ends, or so it seems. Actually, the upstroke (phase II) and the downstroke (phase IV) of the capnogram do not coincide exactly with inspiration and expiration (examine Figures 2.2 and 2.3). During the end of an inspiration, fresh gas that fills the trachea and bronchi does not participate in gas exchange. This fresh gas still fills the trachea when inspiration turns into expiration. Before phase II can be inscribed, therefore, the last gas inhaled and not participating in gas exchange during the previous breath must be expelled. Similarly, fresh gas must sweep away the gas containing carbon dioxide, which still resides in the Y piece from the last expiration. The beginnings of the upstrokes and downstrokes of the capnogram, therefore, are not

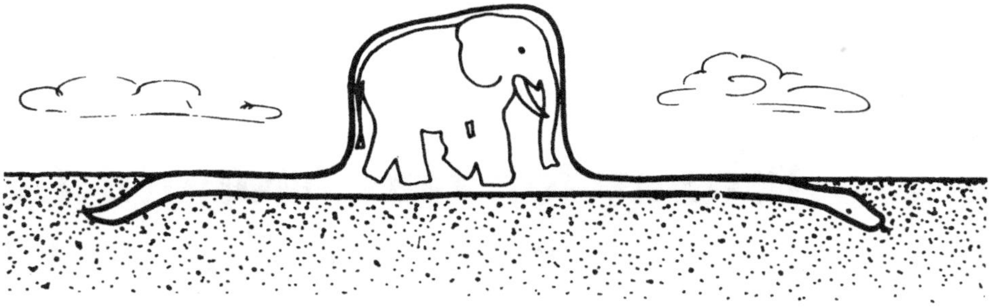

FIGURE 2.1 *A capnogram resembles the silhouette of a snake that has just swallowed an elephant. The image has been called a "capnophant." (Reproduced with permission from Gravenstein JS, Paulus DA, Hayes TJ: Capnography in clinical practice. Stoneham, MA: Butterworths, 1989:11.)*

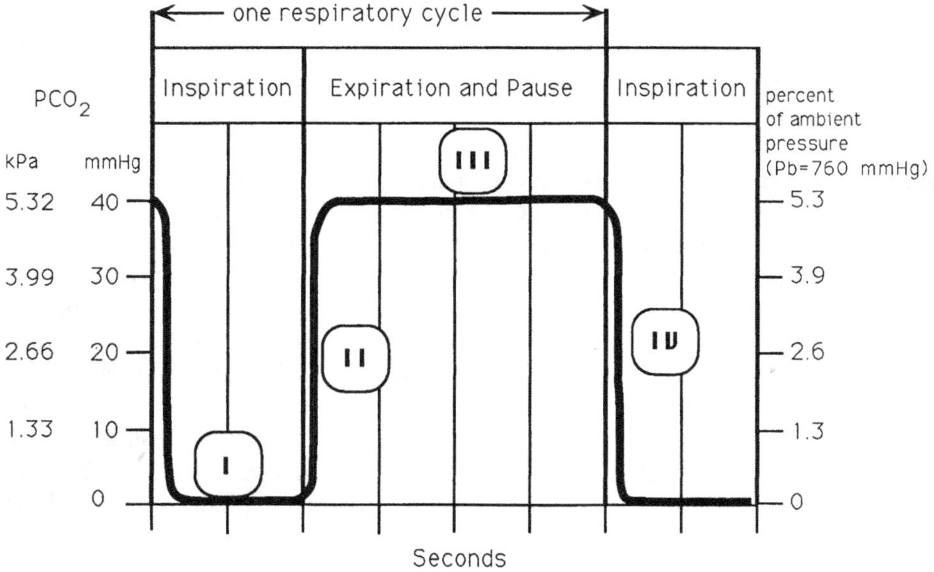

FIGURE 2.2 *The capnogram has four phases: I, inspiration; II, the appearance of carbon dioxide during early expiration; III, the plateau phase, with or without a respiratory pause; and IV, the descending slope of the inspiratory phase. With a respiratory rate of 10 breaths/min, one respiratory cycle would last 6 sec. The ratio of inspiration to expiration is assumed to be 1:2. Gases are assumed to be dry; barometric pressure (Pb) is 760 mm Hg. PCO_2 denotes partial pressure of carbon dioxide.*

synchronous with the initiation of gas movement, but the difference is clinically insignificant.

Beside the fact that the upstrokes and downstrokes of the capnogram fail to signal the exact beginnings of expiration and inspiration, respectively, the time for the gas

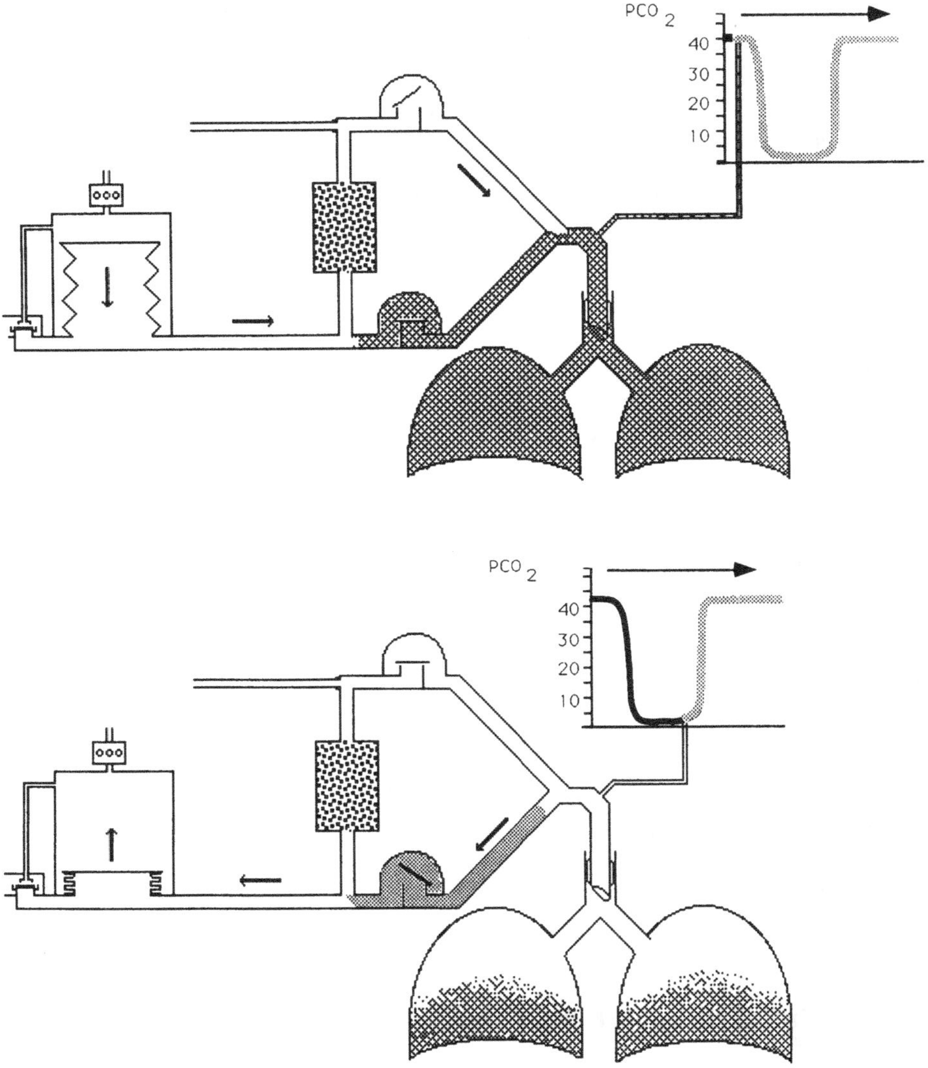

FIGURE 2.3 *A circle breathing system during early inspiration, when carbon dioxide* (shaded area) *still resides in the Y piece, endotracheal tube, and upper airways* (top) *and, of course, in the expiratory branch of the breathing circuit. The capnogram shows end-tidal values. During early expiration, fresh gas still fills the upper airways, endotracheal tube, and Y piece. There is still carbon dioxide in the expiratory tube, left over from the previous breath* (bottom). *The heavy line in the capnogram indicates the part of the curve already recorded; the stippled line is the part to be recorded as ventilation progresses.* PCO_2 *denotes partial pressure of carbon dioxide.*

to travel from sampling port to capnograph in sidestream analyzers delays the signal by a second or two (more about that in Chapter 15).

People who live in a submarine, where the removal of all carbon dioxide taxes the resources, must tolerate a fractional concentration of carbon dioxide in inspired gas ($FICO_2$) of 0.01. We all inhale carbon dioxide when caught in a poorly ventilated room with many other people, all of whom (at least the adults) add at least 200 ml of carbon dioxide per minute to the air they breathe. Some anesthetists like to add carbon dioxide to the atmosphere the patient is breathing after hyperventilation, or to stimulate ventilation (rarely indicated, as a patient not breathing well will have a high partial pressure of carbon dioxide in arterial blood [$PaCO_2$] by definition), or to maintain a normal $PaCO_2$ while inducing hyperventilation in the patient in order to hasten the removal of an inhalation anesthetic.[2]

The capnogram does not always look like the silhouette of a snake that has swallowed an elephant. Sometimes phase II is slanted, phase III slopes or has ripples or clefts, or phase IV is prolonged. Deviations from the ideal call for an analysis of the mechanism that is distorting the capnogram (Figure 2.4).

Capnograms obtained under clinical conditions do not look as neat as experimentally generated capnograms. Spontaneous breathing is rarely machinelike, and mechanical ventilation can be interrupted by artifacts introduced from the outside or by a motion, sigh, or spontaneous breath on the part of the patient. Weinger and Brimm studied postoperative patients and found, probably not unexpectedly, that the highest end-tidal carbon dioxide concentration ($PETCO_2$) from several consecutive breaths gave the best estimation of $PaCO_2$.[3] The authors also observed that in general, the largest spontaneous breaths reflected $PaCO_2$ better than mechanical breaths.

When the patient repeatedly interrupts the mechanical breaths with a brief inspiratory effort (a "breathlet") the anesthetist must determine whether the patient is gasping because of pain (anesthesia too light), hypoventilation (inadequate effective alveolar ventilation), or malfunction of the equipment, or whether a hiccup caused the disturbance. It is poor technique to suppress breathlets with a muscle relaxant without having completed a proper differential diagnosis. The breathlets that regularly dent the smooth plateau of phase III of the capnogram have a typical appearance (Figure 2.5).

OXYGRAPHY AND ANESTHETIGRAPHY

The ability to generate curves that show the changes in concentrations of oxygen, anesthetic vapors, and other gases in respired gas during a respiratory cycle is new. Therefore, new words are needed to describe the activity of generating such curves (______*graphy*), the instrument that measures the gases and generates the curves (______*graphs*), and the curves themselves (______*grams*). The terms *oxygraphy, oxygraph, oxygram,* and *anesthetigraphy, anesthetigraph, anesthetigram* are constructions modeled after the well-established words *capnography, capnograph,* and *capnogram,* which describe parallel activities for carbon dioxide monitoring.

What has been said about the difference between actual and recorded change in carbon dioxide could be repeated for oxygen and anesthetic agents. The beginning of gas flow will not coincide with the onset of the upstroke or downstroke of the oxygram or the anesthetigram. While the capnogram shows higher values during expiration than

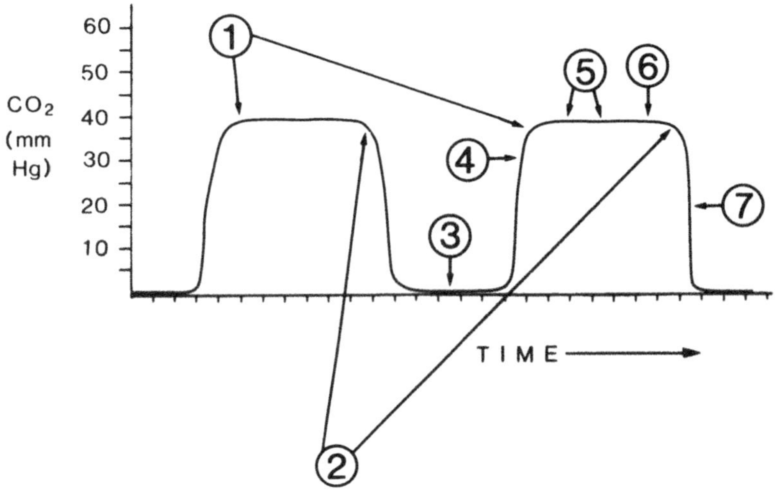

FIGURE 2.4 *The checklist for a capnogram (reproduced with permission from Gravenstein JS, Paulus DA, Hayes TJ: Capnography in clinical practice. Stoneham, MA: Butterworths, 1989):*

1. *Plateau/onset*
   Is there a pattern giving evidence of ventilation?
2. *Plateau/peak*
   Are peak values appropriate? Are the ventilator settings and the patient's respiratory pattern consistent with the capnogram and capnographic findings?
3. *Baseline*
   Is the inspired carbon dioxide tension zero (normal baseline), or is there evidence of rebreathing (elevated baseline)?
4. *Upstroke*
   Is there evidence of slow exhalation (slanted upstroke)?
5. *Plateau/horizontal*
   Is there evidence of uneven emptying of lungs?
6. *Plateau/smooth*
   Is expiration interrupted by inspiratory efforts?
7. *Downstroke*
   Is the downstroke steep, or is there evidence of slow inspiration or partial rebreathing?

during inspiration, the oxygram shows lower values during expiration than during inspiration, as long as the lungs take up oxygen (Figure 2.6). We can easily arrange for conditions during which the end-tidal concentration of oxygen rises above inspired values. We simply have to fill the lungs with oxygen and switch on the nitrous oxide and note the end-tidal and inspired oxygen percentages (Figure 2.7).

Nitrogen too deserves some attention. Because it does not participate in our metabolism, we tend to ignore it. However, during preoxygenation before induction of anesthesia, we are attempting to replace nitrogen with oxygen. As P_{ETO_2} increases, we

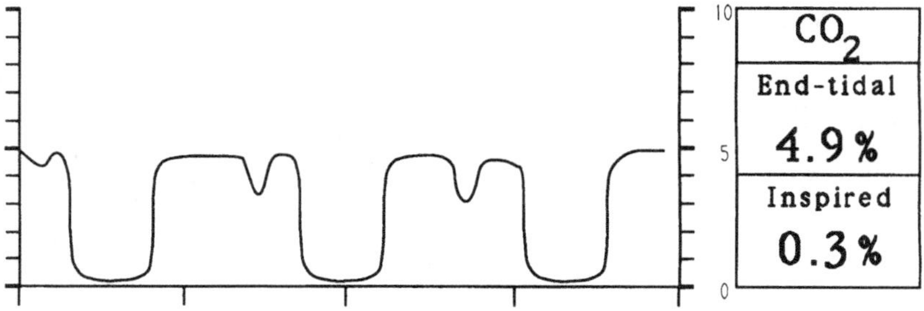

FIGURE 2.5 *Typical appearance of breathlets in a capnogram. The dents in the plateau (phase III) indicate inspiratory efforts by this partially paralyzed patient under general anesthesia with mechanical ventilation. Are the patient's lungs hypoventilated, or is anesthesia too light?*

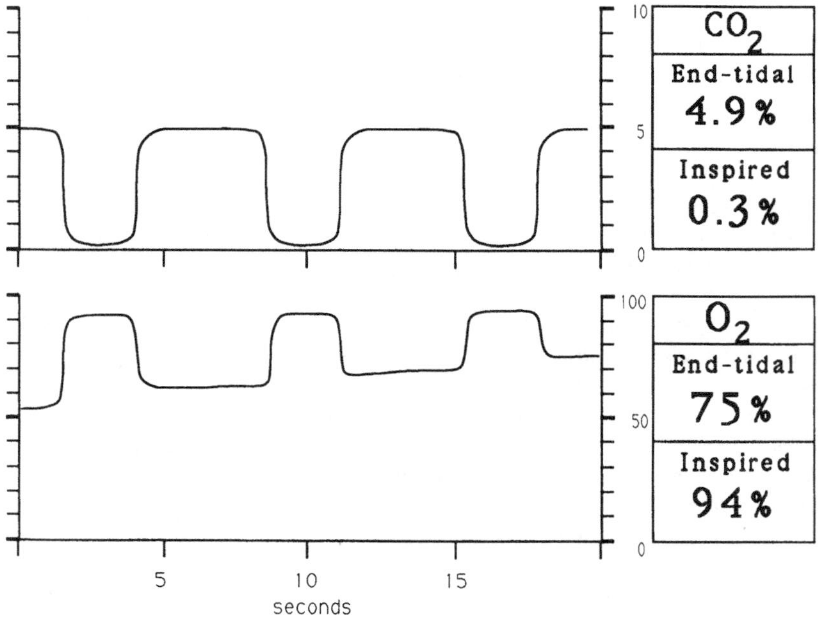

FIGURE 2.6 *Capnogram* (upper trace) *and oxygram* (lower trace) *during the denitrogenation of a patient. Observe the large inspiratory-to-expiratory gradient for oxygen. A circle breathing system is in use.*

may assume that nitrogen decreases. Measuring it in this instance provides redundant information, helpful but not necessary. Nitrogen may appear in the exhaled gas of a patient previously denitrogenated if an air embolism lodges in the lung. When the patient is at risk from air embolism, monitoring nitrogen may support other methods of monitoring for air embolism, including capnography (see also Chapter 14).

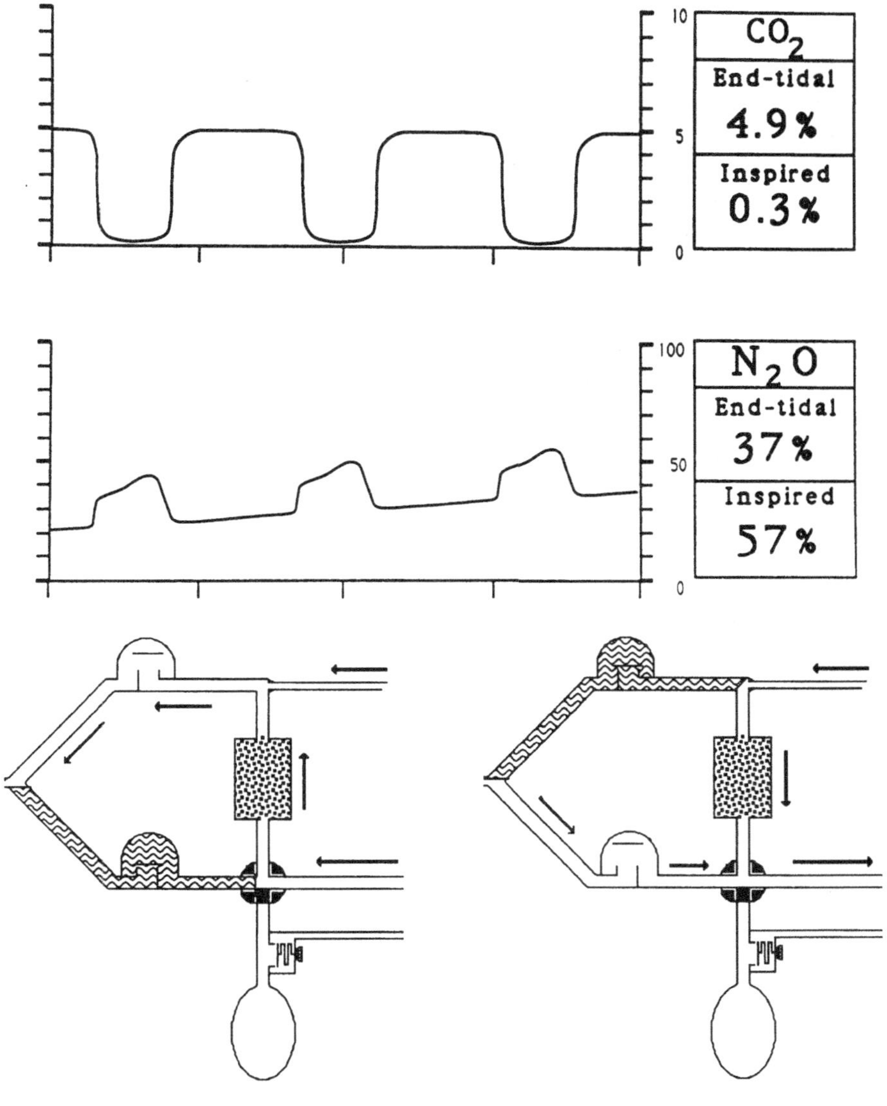

FIGURE 2.7 *Nitrous oxide has been started. The brief peak in the anesthetigram for nitrous oxide just before exhalation is attributed to the properties of the circle breathing system. The breathing circle* (bottom) *has two segments (the inspiratory hose* [left] *and the expiratory hose* [right]) *that conduct gas in one direction only, and one segment that conducts gas in two directions (the absorber and the ventilator and its connecting hose). Gas comes to rest* (shaded area) *in the inspiratory hose whenever the inspiratory valve is closed (during expiration and during the respiratory pause). During that time fresh gas can only flow into the absorber and beyond. The first part of the inspiration, therefore, contains gas left over from the previous breath. The last part of the inspiration contains some fresh gas in addition to the gas that is being rebreathed after having been scrubbed of* CO_2*. See Figure 2.1 for a complete depiction of the breathing circle system.*

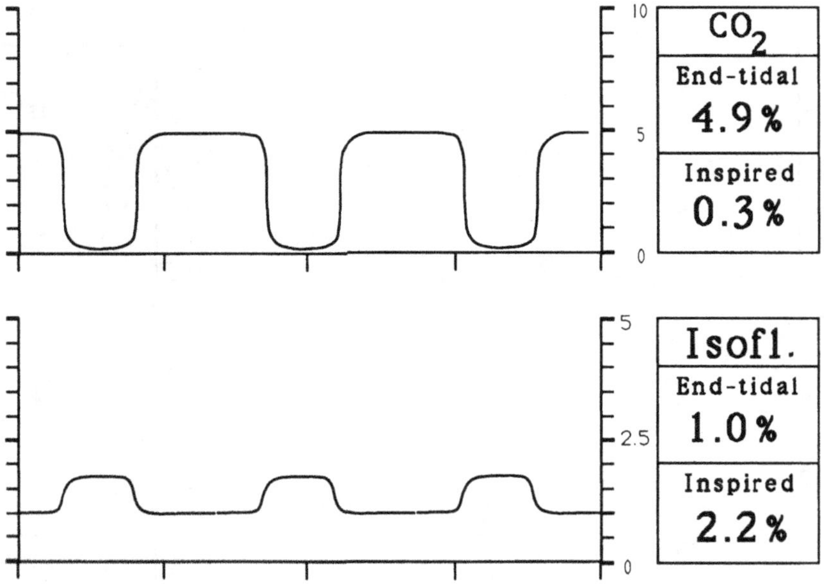

FIGURE 2.8 *Anesthesia with isoflurane (Isoflo) has been underway for 30 min. The inspired concentration of isoflurane exceeds the end-tidal concentration.*

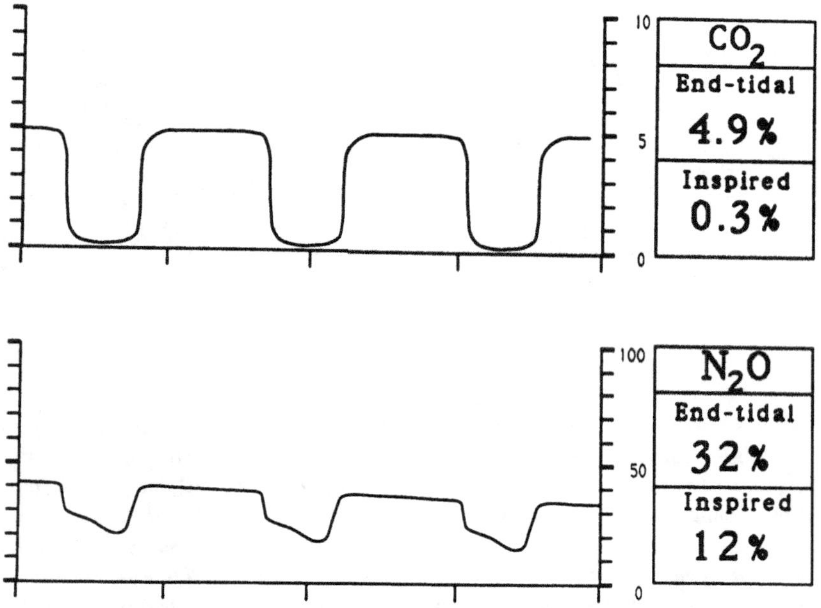

FIGURE 2.9 *At the end of an anesthetic with nitrous oxide, the gas is discontinued and the anesthetigram* (bottom trace) *assumes the shape of a capnogram as nitrous oxide leaves the body with the expired gas. Because a circle breathing system was used, some nitrous oxide returns in the inspired gas. A high flow of fresh gas would reduce nitrous oxide in the inspired gas and hasten the patient's recovery.*

Anesthetigrams vary in appearance according to the phase of anesthesia. While the patient's lungs take up anesthetic, inspiratory values exceed end-tidal values (Figure 2.8). Once gases equilibrate between blood, alveolar gas, and breathing circuit, inspired and end-tidal concentrations are identical. During emergence from anesthesia, when inspired gas contains less anesthetic than end-tidal gas, the anesthetigram assumes the shape of a capnogram (Figure 2.9). Trend plots (Figure 2.10) generated

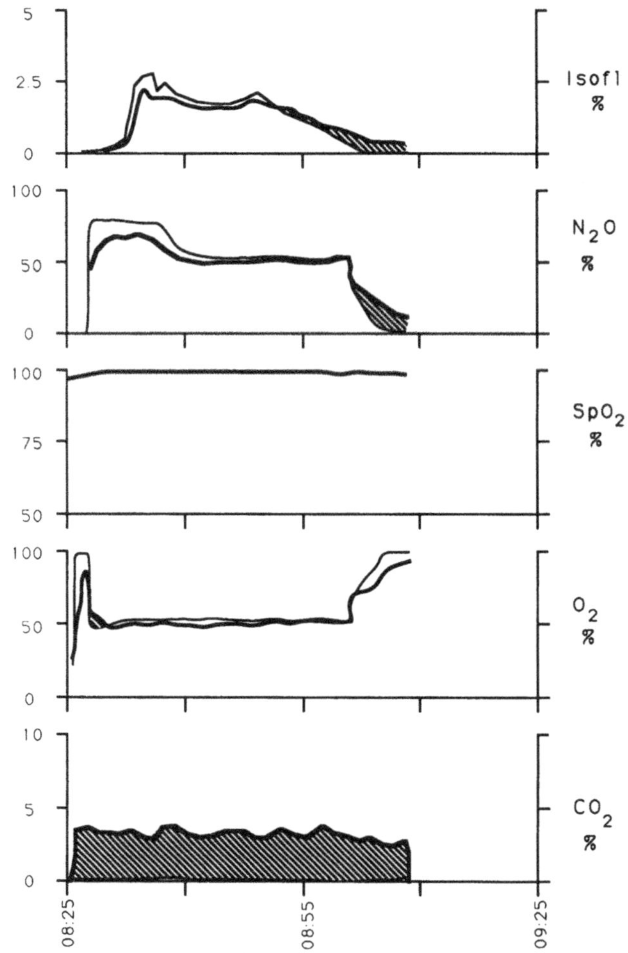

FIGURE 2.10 *A trend plot of an isoflurane (Isofl)–nitrous oxide–oxygen anesthetic. After denitrogenation with oxygen, nitrous oxide and then isoflurane were started. Observe the wash-in and wash-out of oxygen and nitrous oxide at the beginning and end of anesthesia. The trend plots of anesthetigrams, oxygram, and capnogram show inspired as well as end-tidal values. At times, end-tidal values exceed inspired values* (shaded areas on curves). *Observe the large difference between inspired and end-tidal nitrous oxide and oxygen concentrations during induction of and emergence from anesthesia, and how inspired and end-tidal borders cross over as oxygen and nitrous oxide are taken up by the lungs or exhaled. SpO_2 denotes saturation of hemoglobin with oxygen.*

at the end of anesthesia show an overview of the changing concentrations of oxygen and anesthetic in inspired and end-tidal gases. Trend plots permit a useful review of the entire clinical course at the end of anesthesia. Deviations from normal can be identified. In institutions with formal programs for assessing the quality of anesthetic care, summary trend plots may prove valuable.

PULSE OXIMETRY

The pulse oximeter estimates the saturation of hemoglobin with oxygen in peripheral arterial blood (SpO_2). The many instruments, probes, and papers describing pulse oximetry attest to the popularity of this new method of monitoring.[4] The pulse oximeter depends on pulsatile perfusion of the tissue, so the instrument doubles as a monitor of perfusion in addition to monitoring SpO_2.[5] A typical plethysmogram is generated by a pulse oximeter (Figure 2.11). Because the instrument must be calibrated at the factory, the clinician cannot adjust the monitor, and the accuracy of the pulse oximeter leaves much to be desired. Pulse oximeters are excellent trend recorders,

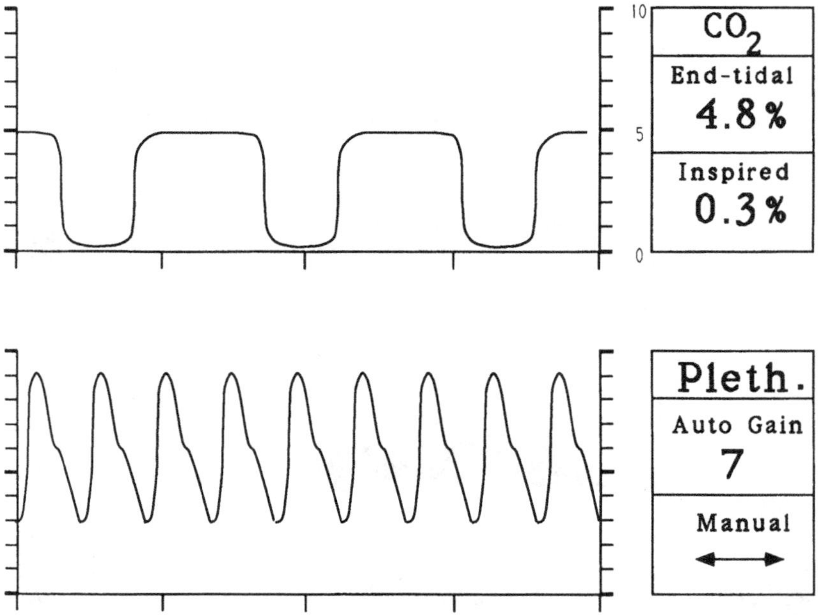

FIGURE 2.11 *The plethysmogram (Pleth.) is plotted on an arbitrary scale. The gain factor was automatically adjusted to 7 arbitrary units. Some monitors enable the user to fix the gain factor; then the monitor still adjusts the baseline but not the gain factor. This permits the clinician to observe changes in the plethysmogram—for example, decreases in the peaks during mechanical inspiration in a hypovolemic patient.*

though, and can alert the clinician to a decreasing SpO_2 long before cyanosis develops.

Between 80% and 100% SpO_2, accuracy with many instruments is no better than ±4% (95% confidence limit); below 80% saturation, it is much worse. Of course, once hemoglobin is fully saturated, the pulse oximeter fails to give information on the partial pressure of oxygen in arterial blood (PaO_2). Between 80% and about 99% SpO_2, PaO_2 can be estimated, depending on the many factors that affect the relationship of PaO_2 to percent saturation (more about that in Chapter 16).

REFERENCES

1. Fletcher R: On-line expiratory carbon dioxide monitoring. Int J Clin Monit Comput 1986; 3:155–163
2. Razis PA: Carbon dioxide—a survey of its use in anesthesia in the United Kingdom. Anaesthesia 1988; 44:348–351
3. Weinger MB, Brimm JE: End-tidal carbon dioxide as a measure of arterial carbon dioxide during intermittent mandatory ventilation. J Clin Monit 1987; 3:73–79
4. Kelleher JF: Pulse oximetry. J Clin Monit 1989; 5:37–62
5. Houagim AR, Backus WW, Manecke G, et al: Pulse oximetry and patient positioning: A report of eight cases. Anesthesiology 1989; 71:454–456

Chapter 3

The Water Vapor Story

In capnometry, much confusion has been caused by the fact that water vapor occupies space in the lungs but most capnometers do not measure water vapor. Inspired gas may be quite dry or may contain little or much water vapor. Expired gas is moist close to the mouth but cools after leaving the airway; thus water vapor condenses and partial pressure of water vapor falls.

Because a misconception of what the analyzer reports may cause consternation about or even errors in interpretation, we should briefly discuss the problem. First, a word about the conventions of reporting gas concentrations and pressures.[1] Pressures (or tensions) are usually reported in mm Hg or torr or kPa (Table 3.1). The sum of partial pressures of gases *in the gas phase* must add up to the ambient or barometric pressure (Pb), which at sea level is usually close to 760 mm Hg or 101 kPa.

That the partial pressures of gases *in solution* do not need to add up to barometric pressure may at first seem startling but is quite logical (Table 3.2). Nitrogen does not participate in metabolism. Its partial pressures are the same in arterial and venous blood. When a patient inhales 100% oxygen, the nitrogen is replaced by oxygen in the lungs. After denitrogenation, the alveolar partial pressures of oxygen, carbon dioxide, and water vapor add up to ambient pressure (here, 760 mm Hg). In blood, most oxygen is bound to hemoglobin, with little in solution. Breathing 100% oxygen, therefore, brings relatively little excess oxygen to the periphery, and venous blood is still blue during denitrogenation with oxygen. The sum of the partial pressures of gases in venous blood do not add up to ambient pressure (Table 3.2).

Gas in the lungs is saturated with water vapor, and temperature influences water vapor tension (Table 3.3). Normally, at a temperature of 37 °C (98.6 °F), water vapor exerts a pressure of about 47 mm Hg (6.25 kPa). If the ambient barometric pressure hovers around 760 mm Hg (101 kPa), only 713 mm Hg (760 minus 47) is available for the other gases in the alveoli, such as oxygen, carbon dioxide, nitrogen, or (during anesthesia) nitrous oxide and the anesthetic vapors. When reporting gas pressures in the alveoli, we speak of BTPS (for *body temperature* of 37 °C at ambient *pressure* and the gas *saturated* with water vapor). Expressed in volume percent of 760 mm Hg ambient pressure, water vapor occupies 6% of the available gas volume in the lungs. If the ambient pressure were 600 mm Hg on a mountain or in Denver, Colorado, and if body temperature were 37 °C, water vapor would still exert 47 mm Hg partial

Table 3.1 Conversion of Torr into kPa

	0	*1*	*2*	*3*	*4*	*5*	*6*	*7*	*8*	*9*
0	0.00	.13	.27	.40	.53	.67	.80	.93	1.06	1.20
10	1.33	1.46	1.60	1.73	1.86	2.00	2.13	2.26	2.39	2.53
20	2.66	2.79	2.93	3.06	3.19	3.33	3.46	3.59	3.72	3.86
30	3.99	4.12	4.26	4.39	4.52	4.66	4.79	4.92	5.05	5.19
40	5.32	5.45	5.59	5.72	5.85	5.99	6.12	6.25	6.38	6.52
50	6.65	6.78	6.92	7.05	7.18	7.32	7.45	7.58	7.71	7.85
60	7.98	8.11	8.25	8.38	8.51	8.65	8.78	8.91	9.04	9.18
70	9.31	9.44	9.58	9.71	9.84	9.98	10.11	10.24	10.37	10.51
80	10.64	10.77	10.91	11.04	11.17	11.31	11.44	11.57	11.70	11.84
90	11.97	12.10	12.24	12.37	12.50	12.64	12.77	12.90	13.03	13.17
100	13.30	13.43	13.57	13.70	13.83	13.97	14.10	14.23	14.36	14.50
110	14.63	14.76	14.90	15.03	15.16	15.30	15.43	15.56	15.69	15.83
120	15.96	16.09	16.23	16.36	16.49	16.63	16.76	16.89	17.02	17.16
130	17.29	17.42	17.56	17.69	17.82	17.96	18.09	18.22	18.35	18.49
140	18.62	18.75	18.89	19.02	19.15	19.29	19.42	19.55	19.68	19.82
150	19.95	20.08	20.22	20.35	20.48	20.62	20.75	20.88	21.01	21.15
160	21.28	21.41	21.55	21.68	21.81	21.95	22.08	22.21	22.34	22.48
170	22.61	22.74	22.88	23.01	23.14	23.28	23.41	23.54	23.67	23.81
180	23.94	24.07	24.21	24.34	24.47	24.61	24.74	24.87	25.00	25.14
190	25.27	25.40	25.54	25.67	25.80	25.94	26.07	26.20	26.33	26.47
200	26.60	26.73	26.87	27.00	27.13	27.27	27.40	27.53	27.66	27.80
210	27.93	28.06	28.20	28.33	28.46	28.60	28.73	28.86	28.99	29.13
220	29.26	29.39	29.53	29.66	29.79	29.93	30.06	30.19	30.32	30.46
230	30.59	30.72	30.86	30.99	31.12	31.26	31.39	31.52	31.65	31.79
240	31.92	32.05	32.19	32.32	32.45	32.59	32.72	32.85	32.98	33.12
250	33.25	33.38	33.52	33.65	33.78	33.92	34.05	34.18	34.31	34.45
260	34.58	34.71	34.85	34.98	35.11	35.25	35.38	35.51	35.64	35.78
270	35.91	36.04	36.18	36.31	36.44	36.58	36.71	36.84	36.97	37.11
280	37.24	37.37	37.51	37.64	37.77	37.91	38.04	38.17	38.30	38.44
290	38.57	38.70	38.84	38.97	39.10	39.24	39.37	39.50	39.63	39.77
300	39.90	40.03	40.17	40.30	40.43	40.57	40.70	40.83	40.96	41.10

To convert torr (mm Hg) into kPa, find torr value on left margin and top line. The $PaCO_2$ of 42 mm Hg is 5.59 kPa.

Source: Gravenstein JJ, Paulus DA. Clinical monitoring practice. Philadelphia: J.B. Lippincott, 1987: 46–47. With permission of the publisher.

pressure. This is because vapor pressure varies with temperature but not with the presence or absence of other gases or with atmospheric pressure. At an ambient pressure of 600 mm Hg, water vapor pressure of 47 mm Hg would occupy almost 8% volume of the lung's gas volume.

Table 3.2 Partial Pressures of Respiratory Gases under Different Conditions

	mm Hg					kPa				
Patient with core temperature of 37.1°C	PO_2	PCO_2	PN_2	PH_2O	*Sum of Partial Pressures*	PO_2	PCO_2	PN_2	PH_2O	*Sum of Partial Pressures*
Patient breathing room air										
Artery	100	40	573	47	760	13.3	5.3	76.2	6.2	101
Central vein	46	46	573	47	712	6.1	6.1	76.2	6.2	94.6
Patient breathing 100% oxygen										
Artery	673	40	0	47	760	89.1	5.3	0	6.2	101
Central vein	50	46	0	47	137	6.7	6.1	0	6.2	19

Table 3.3 Pressure of Water Vapor at Different Temperatures

Temperature		
°C	*°F*	*Vapor Pressure (mm Hg)*
20	68.0	17.4
25	77.0	23.7
26	78.8	25.2
27	80.6	26.7
28	82.4	28.3
29	84.2	30.0
30	86.0	31.5
31	87.8	33.7
32	89.6	35.6
33	91.4	37.7
34	93.2	39.8
35	95.0	41.8
36	96.8	44.2
37	98.6	46.6
38	100.4	49.3
39	102.2	52.0
40	104.0	54.9
41	105.8	58.3
42	107.6	61.5
43	109.4	64.8
44	111.2	68.2

Fresh gas delivered by the central gas supply or cylinders of an anesthesia machine is said to be "bone dry." The concentration of dry gases is often expressed in percent or fraction (F), where 100% is equivalent to an F of 1.0. The oxygen (FO_2) in dry air, therefore, is 0.209. In clinical practice the condition is specified as STPD (standard temperature [0 °C], pressure [760 mm Hg], dry). In all anesthesia systems, bone-dry gas is delivered into the breathing circuit. The inhaled gas in circle systems, however, is not bone dry, because some of the inhaled gas contains water vapor (the amount depends on temperature) from the previously exhaled breath and from the carbon dioxide absorber. Sometimes we employ humidifiers that warm the inspired gas and add to it water droplets or water vapor. In these systems, the water vapor pressure in the inspired gas depends on fresh gas flow (FGF), tidal volume, the efficacy of the humidifier, and the temperature of the inspired gas.

Assume that we use a Mapleson rebreathing system (Figure 3.1) and that we are running 4 L/min oxygen and 6 L/min nitrous oxide. At a barometric pressure of 760 mm Hg, the FO_2 in the inspired dry gas would be 0.4 or 40% of 760 mm Hg, or 304.0 mm Hg; the FN_2O would be 0.6 or 60% of 760 mm Hg, or 456.0 mm Hg. As the patient inhales this mixture, the gas is warmed and becomes saturated with water vapor. In the alveoli (before adding carbon dioxide or absorbing oxygen or nitrous

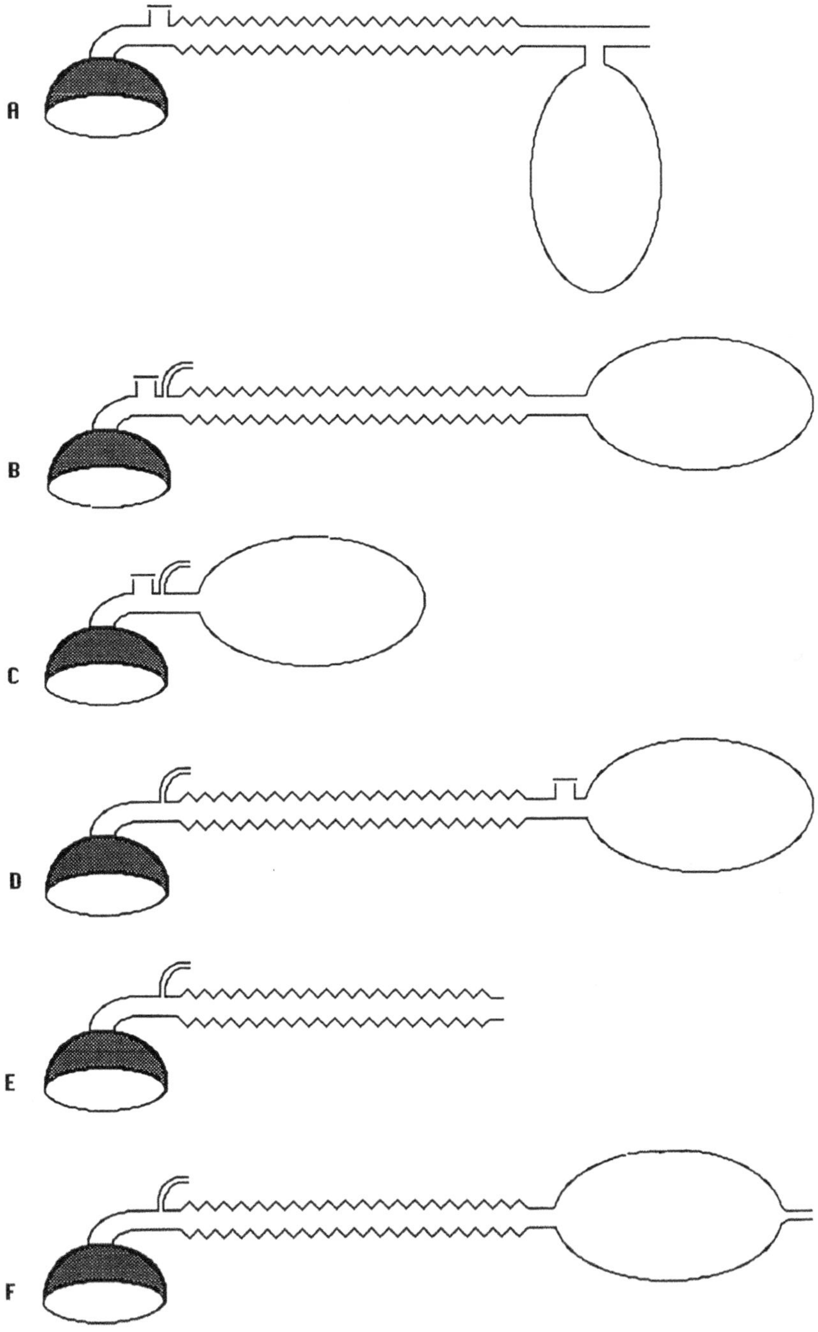

FIGURE 3.1 *Anesthesia breathing systems, classified A through F by Mapleson. The nomenclature suggested by Mapleson has been widely adopted to describe the different arrangements of fresh gas inlet, breathing bag, and relief outlet for excess gas. (Reproduced with permission.[1]) These arrangements have been called T-piece systems or rebreathing systems.*

oxide), the PO_2 would be calculated as $FO_2 \times (P_b - 47)$. With $P_b = 760$ mm Hg, PO_2 would now be 285.2 mm Hg. A similar calculation for nitrous oxide yields a PN_2O of 427.8 mm Hg. Thus, the addition of water vapor in the lungs would have reduced the percentage of oxygen from 40% to 37.5% and the percentage of nitrous oxide from 60% to 56.3%. Water vapor must be taken into account when partial pressure of inspired oxygen is compared with PaO_2.

Clinicians have worried about the loss of water in expired gas. The more humid the inspired gas, the less water the body will have to contribute to saturate gas in the lungs and, thus, the less water and heat the body will lose. The higher the FGF and, thus, the drier the inspired gas, the more water will be lost by the body. In circle breathing systems, water vapor and temperature in inspired gas increase over time, more so with low than with high FGFs. Marked differences may occur, depending on the FGF after 120 min (Table 3.4).[2] With the Bain system, inspired gas tends to be drier than with a circle system.[3]

Regardless of the system employed, exhaled gas leaves the alveoli fully saturated with water vapor. This gas cools as it leaves the mouth or the endotracheal tube, and some of the water vapor begins to condense. Then the gas continues its travels outside the body and soon assumes the temperature of the room or of the analyzer. As the water vapor pressure drops, the partial pressures available for the other gases (oxygen, nitrous oxide, carbon dioxide, anesthetic agents) increase.

What should the gas monitoring instrument report?[4] The instruments are calibrated with dry gas of known FCO_2. However, the gas presented to the instrument for analysis may be dry or more or less diluted by water vapor. Sidestream analyzers usually manage to reduce water vapor in the gas samples to a humidity that comes close to that of room air. In mainstream (on-airway) analyzers, the expired gas is assumed to be saturated with water vapor, and the inspired gas to have a low concentration of water vapor. If the instruments could determine the concentration of water vapor in the sample, a suitable algorithm would enable them to report accurate data. But the water vapor content is not measured. The corrections, therefore, are approximations.

The options include reporting all gases as if they were dry and as they exist in the fresh gas, reporting all gases as if they were saturated with water vapor at 37 °C and as they exist in the lungs, or reporting gases as a combination of these.

Reporting the partial pressure of all inspired and end-tidal gases as if they were at BTPS permits comparisons of pressures of arterial or mixed venous blood gases with pressures of respired gases without requiring conversion of the values. To explain differences between the reported respired gases and arterial or mixed venous gases, for example, owing to a ventilation-perfusion mismatch, correction for water vapor would be unnecessary. A disadvantage would be that the sum of all partial pressures of inspired dry gases would not add up to ambient pressure, because BTPS would assume the presence of water vapor pressure at the patient's temperature. Consequently, even pure oxygen would be reported as 93.8 volume percent, or 713 mm Hg at BTPS, when the ambient pressure is 760 mm Hg and the patient's temperature is 37.1 °C. A strong argument can be made for reporting end-tidal gas at BTPS, as the expired gas arrives laden with water vapor, which then progressively condenses.

Table 3.4 Fresh Gas Flow in Circle Breathing System

	Gas Flow (L/min)		
	0.6	*3.0*	*6.0*
Absolute inspiratory humidity after 120 min (mg H_2O/L)	21	15	14
Inspiratory temperature after 120 min (°C)	32	26	25

Rounded data from Kleeman PP: Klimatisierung anaesthetischer Gase durch Reduktion des Frischgasflows. In: Jantzen J-PAH, Kleemann PP, eds. Narkosebeatmung: Low flow, minimal flow, Geschlossenes System. Stuttgart, FRG: Schattauer, 1989: 113.

Another choice is to report values for inspired gases as fractions of dry gases and convert the end-tidal values for gases to BTPS. That lets us speak of an FIO_2 of 1.0, when pure oxygen is administered, and end-tidal gas values can be compared with blood gas values without having to correct respired gas values for water vapor.

Another option is to report the fractions of both inspired and end-tidal gases as if they were dry (STPD). That yields consistent data but obliges the clinician to remember water vapor when comparing values from the analysis of respired gases with blood gas values.

Before purchasing a monitoring system, ask how the manufacturer has dealt with the problem of water vapor so that there will be no misunderstanding.

REFERENCES

1. Otis AB: Quantitative relationships in steady state gas exchange. In: Fenn WO, Rahn H, eds. Handbook of physiology, section 3: Respiration, volume 1. Washington DC: American Physiological Society, 1964: 681–698
2. Kleemann PP: Klimatisierung anaesthetischer Gase durch Reduktion des Frischgasflows. In: Jantzen J-PAH, Kleeman PP, eds. Narkosebeatmung. Stuttgart, FRG: Schattauer, 1989
3. Bengtson JP, Bengtson A, Sonander H, et al: Humidity of the Bain and circle systems reassessed. Anesth Analg 1989; 69:83–86
4. Severinghaus JW: Water vapor calibration errors in some capnometers: Respiratory conventions misunderstood by manufacturers? Anesthesiology 1989; 70:996–998

Chapter 4

Of Gas Volumes, Flows, and Time Constants

When the anesthetist sets the flowmeters for oxygen and nitrous oxide to 1 L/min and 2 L/min, respectively, and sets the vaporizer to deliver 1% of an inhalation anesthetic, what can the patient's inspired gas be expected to contain? Only in the tubing carrying the fresh gas to the anesthesia breathing system (shaded tubing in Figure 4.1) will the gas composition reflect the settings of the flowmeters and the vaporizer, provided they are correctly calibrated. But even here surprises are in store. When not in use, the vaporizer will contain anesthetic liquid and, depending on its vapor pressure and the ambient temperature, more or less anesthetic vapor. Therefore, with some vaporizers, when first opening the device, this stored anesthetic vapor will be released suddenly and a surge of anesthetic vapor will be discharged into the breathing circuit (Philip JH: Personal communication, 1990). From then on, a properly calibrated vaporizer will deliver the selected percentage. Some vaporizers are flow dependent, that is, at very low flow rates the vaporizer may not deliver the set percentage of vapor. Read the manufacturer's description of the vaporizer to learn the best FGF for accurate metering of anesthetic vapor.

When the gas enters the breathing system, matters become quite complex. The fresh gases mix with the gas already contained in the breathing system. The tubing of the breathing system and the carbon dioxide absorber may absorb some of the anesthetic. The patient absorbs some of the inspired gas and adds at least carbon dioxide. The end-tidal gas, therefore, does not resemble the inspired gas, and the inspired gas does not resemble the fresh gas. Anesthetists who can monitor inspired and end-tidal gas concentrations need not worry. They can adjust the flow rate of the gases and the vaporizer setting until the inspired or end-tidal concentrations have reached the desired levels.

The rate at which we can replace a gas in the breathing system with a fresh gas depends on the flow rate of the fresh gas. If we have a breathing system that contains 7 L of air (a 3-L reservoir bag, a 2-L carbon dioxide absorber, and breathing hoses and connecting tubing that hold 2 L), and if we flow 100 ml of oxygen into the system, it will take a long time to replace all the air with oxygen. If we instead flow 100 L

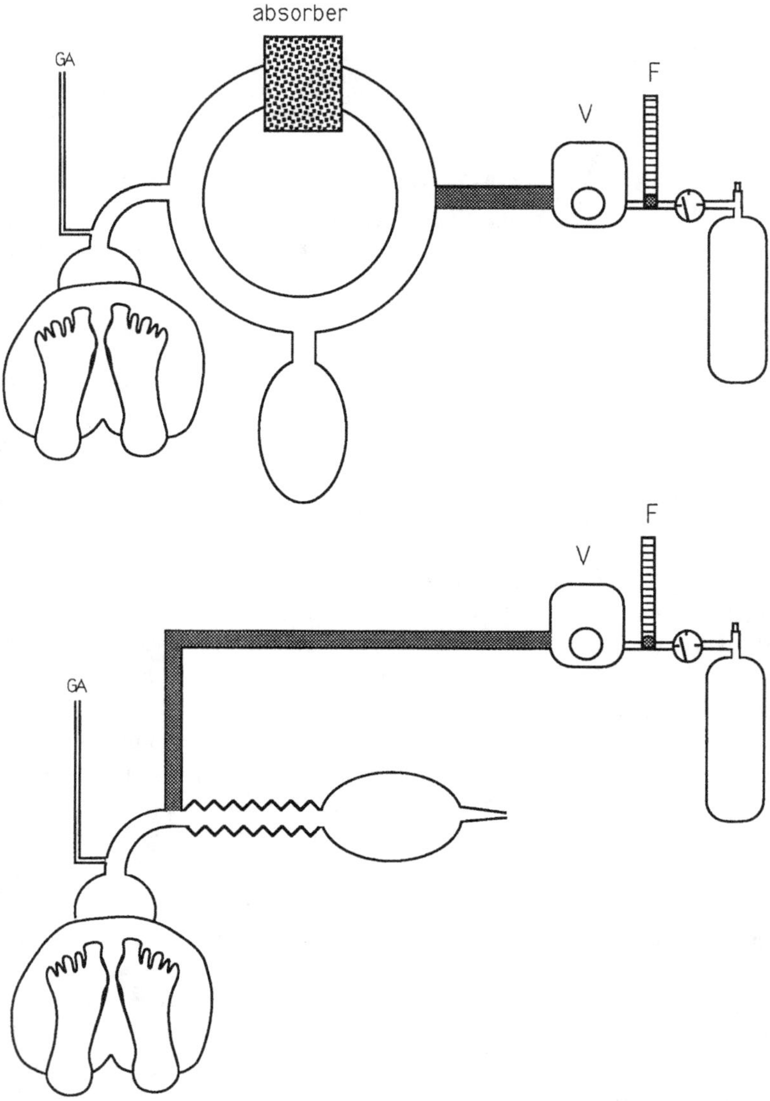

FIGURE 4.1 *The settings of the flow meter (F) and vaporizer (V) determine the composition of the fresh gas. Once the gas emerges from the supply hose for fresh gas* (shaded tubing), *the gas composition is affected by the breathing circuit and the patient (here, viewed from below). Shown are the outlines of a circle system as a reminder of its large volumes, and a Mapleson system as a reminder that rebreathing will affect gas composition. It is possible to monitor the concentrations of inspired and end-tidal gases close to the patient's mouth (GA denotes capillary to gas analyzer) but difficult to predict those concentrations without measurements.*

of oxygen into it, it will take very little time. We can use the concept of time constants to calculate the time required to replace one gas in a system with another gas.[1]

First, consider the example of a vessel containing 10 L of water (Figure 4.2). We

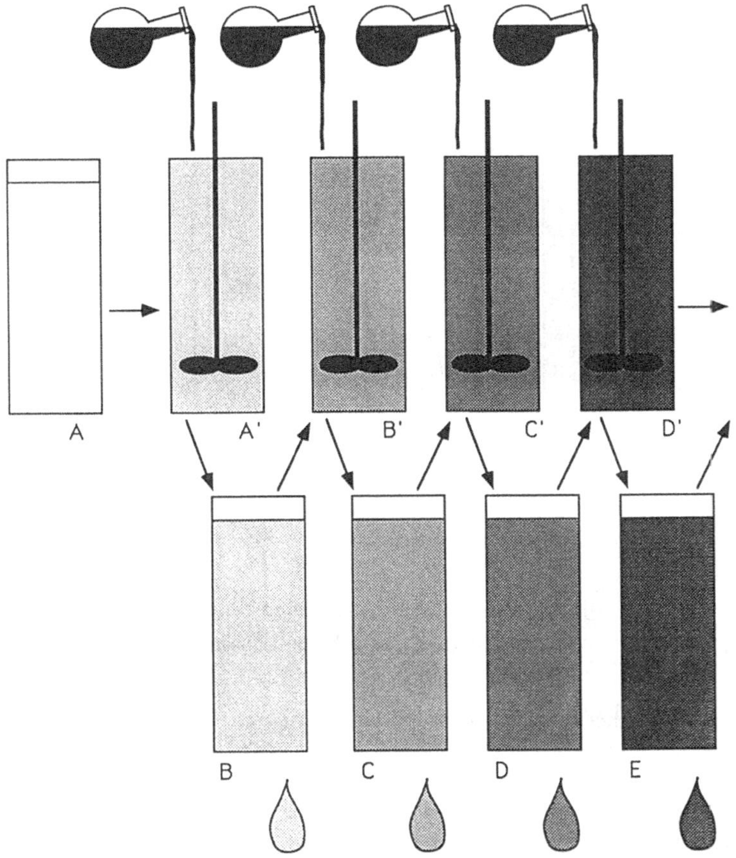

FIGURE 4.2 *The time-constant concept. Vessel A contains 10 L of water. We add 1 L of ink and stir (A'), then drain off 1 L to obtain B. The water becomes more and more inky as we repeat the process. After the tenth liter of ink has been added, the water will contain 63% ink. The time it takes to accomplish this is called a time constant. After four time constants, the vessel will contain 98.2% ink.*

add 1 L of ink, mix it, and then drain off 1 L of water (now containing some of the ink). After we have repeated this process 10 times, we will have added a volume of ink equal to that of the vessel, and we will have drained an equal volume. The vessel will now contain 10 L of 63% ink. If we have added a liter of ink every minute, it will have taken 10 min to complete the process. In that case, one time constant would be 10 min. If we had taken 1 day to drip the 10 L of ink, drop by drop, into the vessel containing 10 L of water (with complete mixing after every increment and drainage of the excess so that the volume always remained at 10 L), one time constant would have been 1 day.

Consider the rising concentration of helium (the new gas) in a 7-L anesthesia breathing circuit originally containing air (Figure 4.3). We add the helium in 350-ml increments, assuming instantaneous and complete mixing and removal of 350 ml of the

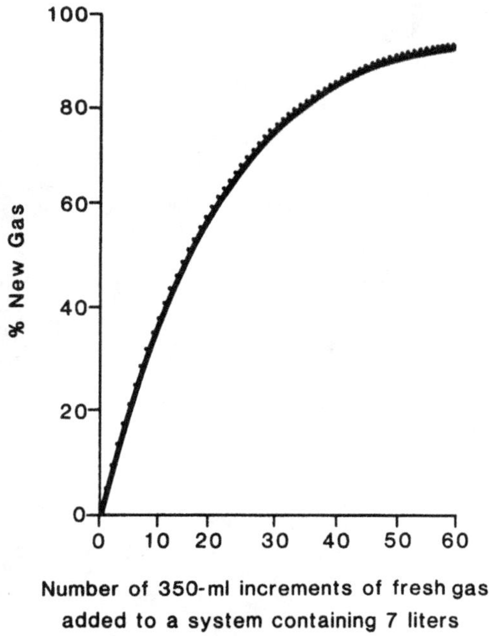

FIGURE 4.3 *Generation of a curve showing the time constant during anesthesia. The curve was prepared by calculating the time required to replace the gas in a 7-L anesthesia system with a new gas. The new gas was added to the system in arbitrarily selected increments of 350 ml. Complete mixing was assumed to have taken place, and excess gas was assumed to have been vented, after mixing. Thus, each point on the abscissa of the curve represents one 350-ml addition of the new gas. The ordinate shows how the new gas gradually replaced the old gas in the system. After one time constant, 63% of the volume had been filled with the new gas. A time constant will be short if the fresh gas is added rapidly. For example, at a flow rate of 7 L/min, the time constant would be 1 min for this 7-L system (20 times 350 ml). The abscissa, therefore, should be viewed as a time axis, the units of which will change with the flow rate of fresh gas. The shape of the curve would be the same whether fresh gas had been added in minute or hour intervals.*

new mixture after each increment. We will have added 7 L of helium after 20 such increments—that is, as much as the original content of the breathing system—and the system will contain 63% helium. If we accomplish this in 1 min by using a flow rate of 7 L/min, the time constant is 1 min. The system would contain 86.5% helium after two time constants and 95.0% and 98.2% helium after three and four time constants, respectively. If we had set the gas flow at 3.5 L/min of helium, one time constant would have been 2 min. The following tabulation shows how the graph was constructed.

1. Start with a system containing 7000 ml of air.
2. Add 350 ml of helium.

3. Assume instantaneous mixing.
4. Spill 350 ml in order to reestablish a 7000-ml volume. The spilled gas will contain a mixture of helium and air (4.76% of the added helium and 4.76% of the original air will have been spilled).
5. The 7-L volume now contains 6666.67 ml of air and 333.33 ml of helium.
6. With the second and subsequent increments, repeat the maneuver.

After 20 increments (equal to the original volume of the system), the breathing system will contain 63% helium. The time required to reach that point will be one time constant. The time constant is often referred to as τ, which can be approximated as follows: $\tau = V/F$, where V (in our example) is the capacity of the breathing circuit (in liters), and F the flow into that circuit (in L/min). The liters cancel and time remains. Scientifically τ can be calculated as $(1 - e^{-1})$ or $(1 - 2.718^{-1})$ or $(1 - 0.37) = 0.63$, the derivation of which I cannot supply.

In our discussion, we have disregarded other factors that influence the rate of change of the anesthetic concentration in the inspired gas, such as absorption of the agents by components of the anesthesia system and by the patient.

Nervous anesthetists often make frequent, small adjustments of the vaporizer in response to a patient's fluctuating blood pressure. Contemplation of the time constants reveals how much impact to expect on the inspired concentration of the anesthetic. With the customary low FGF, little is accomplished with small adjustments of the vaporizer.

Time constants also play a role in the Mapleson system if some gas is being rebreathed. Calculating time constants, however, is impossible without information on the volume of gas being rebreathed. Monitoring gas concentrations in inspired gas makes the calculation unnecessary.

Time constants can be calculated for the lungs as well. The larger the functional residual capacity of the lungs, the larger the time constant; the larger the effective alveolar ventilation, the shorter the time constant. Time constants for the lungs have an additional dimension. Classically, a time constant (expressed in seconds) for the lungs is defined as the product of total lung compliance (in liters per centimeter of water or liters per kilopascal) times pulmonary resistance (centimeters of water per liter per second or kilopascals per liter per second); thus, we work with pressures, volumes, and time, whereas previously we worked with volumes, flow rates, and time. The greater the compliance, the more volume the system will accept before a set pressure is reached; conversely, the greater the resistance, the longer it takes to fill the functional residual capacity with new gas.

Time constants have been reported for tissues also. The ratio of the volume of distribution to the effective blood flow delivering a drug to tissue is called the time constant. The approximate time constant for the vessel-rich group (brain, heart, kidney, and liver) is 3 to 4 min; for the muscle group it is 120 min, and for fat, close to 3000 min.

REFERENCE

1. Eger EI II: Anesthetic uptake and action. Baltimore: Williams and Wilkins, 1976: 78–79

Chapter 5

Solubility

Once the gas anesthetic is delivered to the lungs, ventilation governs how much anesthetic is made available for absorption through the alveolar membrane. The solubility of the anesthetic determines how much of the anesthetic goes into solution in the blood. Cardiac output controls how much anesthetic is carried away in the arterial blood. Tissue blood flow regulates how much is brought into the organs. The volume of the organs and the solubility of the anesthetic in the tissue of the organ, finally, establish how much of the delivered anesthetic goes into solution in any given organ, and in the aggregate, in the body. The compartments of greatest interest are the richly perfused, vessel-rich group, which consists of the parenchymatous organs such as heart, brain, intestines, kidney, and liver; the large muscle group, which is moderately well perfused; and the poorly perfused fat (Figure 5.1). A most instructive computer program presented by Philip enables a novice to change ventilation, cardiac output, fresh gas flow, and anesthetic concentration of different inhalation anesthetics in order to explore how these factors alter the uptake and distribution of inhalation anesthetics.[1]

SOLUBILITY

Solubility of gases or vapors in water, blood, or tissue is usually expressed as a coefficient—that is, as a normalized ratio of water or blood to gas, or of tissue to blood. Two commonly used solubility coefficients are named after their original proponents, Bunsen (equation 5.1) and Ostwald (equation 5.2):

$$\text{alpha} = \frac{\begin{array}{c}\text{volume of gas dissolved in 1 unit volume of water}\\ \text{(at 273 °K absolute temperature)}\end{array}}{\begin{array}{c}\text{volume of gas present in 1 unit volume}\\ \text{of gas at atmospheric pressure}\end{array}} \qquad (5.1)$$

$$\text{lambda} = \frac{\begin{array}{c}\text{volume of gas dissolved in 1 unit volume of water}\\ \text{(at specified temperature)}\end{array}}{\begin{array}{c}\text{volume of gas present in 1 unit volume}\\ \text{of gas at specified partial pressure}\end{array}} \qquad (5.2)$$

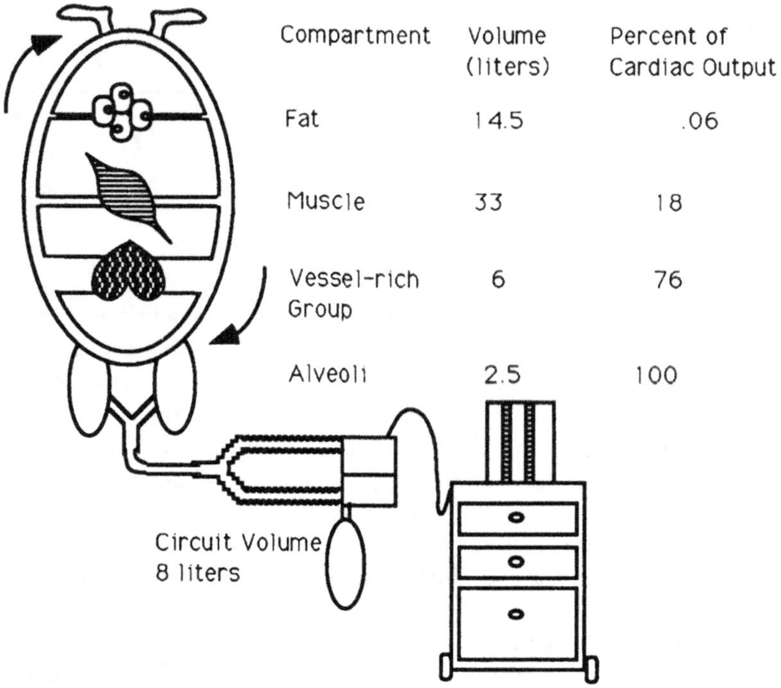

FIGURE 5.1 *An anesthesia machine with its breathing circuit, and a body with its compartments. Observe the large blood supply to the small vessel-rich groups (indicated by the heart, but including brain and intestines), the large muscle group (striated) with a good blood supply, and the fat group with the smallest blood supply.*

The Bunsen coefficient is calculated from an Ostwald solubility coefficient by correcting to standard conditions. The Ostwald coefficient is multiplied by 273 °K, and the product is divided by the temperature (in degrees Kelvin) at which the Ostwald coefficient was measured.

An Ostwald solubility coefficient (lambda) of 5, for example, means that at equilibrium at the given temperature, a given volume of solvent contains five times as much gas as is found in an equal volume of gas overlying the solvent (Table 5.1). In other words, the gas is five times as soluble in the solvent as it is in the gas phase. Because of the large differences between some anesthetics, agents like nitrous oxide and xenon are sometimes called insoluble agents, while ether is called a soluble agent. This convenient labeling both helps and hinders. For example, it helps by drawing attention to the fact that halothane is almost five times as soluble in blood as nitrous oxide; it hinders by obscuring the fact that nitrous oxide is quite soluble in comparison to certain other gases. For instance, nitrous oxide is 33 times as soluble as nitrogen. Indeed, at equilibrium with 70% nitrous oxide, the average adult can hold many liters of nitrous oxide but far less than a liter of nitrogen when in equilibrium with air. At first, it seems

Table 5.1 Ostwald Solubility Coefficients (37°C)

	Blood
Diethyl ether	12
Halothane	2.3
Enflurane	1.8
Isoflurane	1.4
Sevoflurane	0.6
Nitrous oxide	0.47
Desflurane	0.42
Xenon	0.14
Nitrogen*	0.015

Modified with permission from Eger EI II: Anesthetic uptake and action. Baltimore: Williams and Wilkins, 1976:82.

*Not an anesthetic at ambient pressure.

astonishing that many anesthetic gases find comfort, and thus seek residence, in a liquid such as blood rather than dwell among the other gases in the gas phase (Figure 5.2).

When the partial pressure of a gas is increased, more gas is forced into solution, but the ratio between volumes of gas in the solvent and gas in the gas phase stays the same, as long as temperature remains constant. The partial pressure of the gas does not influence the Ostwald solubility coefficient. Temperature, however, does: the higher the temperature, the lower the solubility.

Given the different solubility coefficients of anesthetic agents, we must expect differences when we use a soluble or a relatively insoluble agent. Assume that a patient inhales 2% nitrous oxide one time and 2% halothane another time. If each time over 1 min we bring 5 L of gas into contact with alveoli perfused, ideally, with 5 L of blood, the patient removes far more halothane than nitrous oxide from the alveoli, because at equilibrium blood contains 2.3 volume units of halothane compared with only 0.47 volume units of nitrous oxide. If so little nitrous oxide is taken up by the blood, the expired gas contains much nitrous oxide, whereas much halothane is taken up by the blood. The expired gas contains little halothane.

Many years ago, Severinghaus[2] used an electrical analog to demonstrate how the inspired concentration of an anesthetic approaches the alveolar concentration of the agent; he also illustrated how solubility influences the rate of equilibration (Figure 5.3). In a similar, computer-generated plot, Eger showed that ventilation affects the approach of inspired to alveolar concentration (Figure 5.4). The uptake of soluble agents is accelerated with hyperventilation, more so than that of less soluble agents. Conversely, pushing more blood through the lungs to carry away anesthetic also accelerates the uptake of the drug, more so with soluble agents than with less soluble agents, as they are already rapidly approaching equilibrium (Figure 5.5).

With the Gas Man® computer program, we can demonstrate the effects of variations in cardiac output, ventilation, or FGF on the distribution of an anesthetic, for example nitrous oxide (Figure 5.6), in different compartments of the body. Reducing

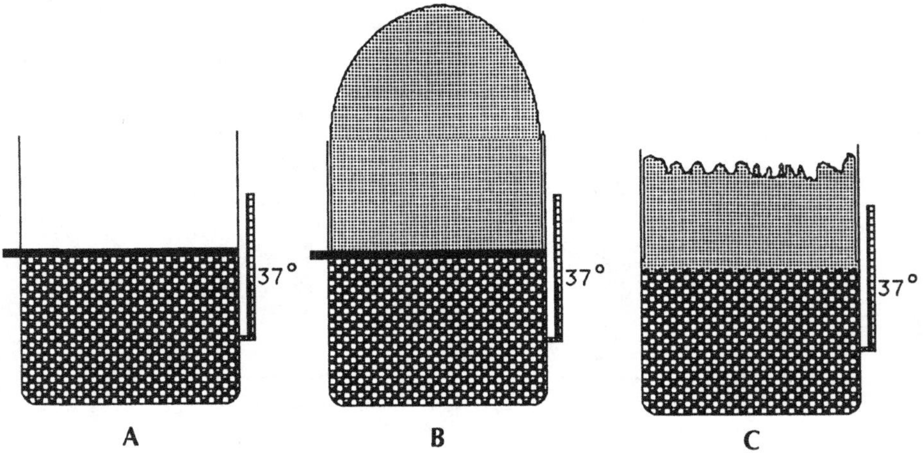

FIGURE 5.2 *The solubility of anesthetic agents in blood. In bottle A, blood at 37°C is kept under a black lid. In bottle B, a balloon filled with nitrous oxide at 1 atmosphere of pressure has been placed on top of the black lid. In bottle C, the lid separating blood from nitrous oxide has been removed, and the gas can equilibrate with the blood; soon, much of the gas will have dissolved in the blood. The partial pressure of the gas in the remaining balloon is the same as it was before and the same as the partial pressure of the gas in the blood: 1 atmosphere. But the volume of the balloon has shrunk because much of the gas has dissoved in the blood. Measuring the ratio of gas volumes in the blood and in the gas phase, we find that the ratio of volume dissolved to the volume in gas phase is as 1 is to 0.47. The solubility coefficient of nitrous oxide in blood at 37°C is 0.47.*

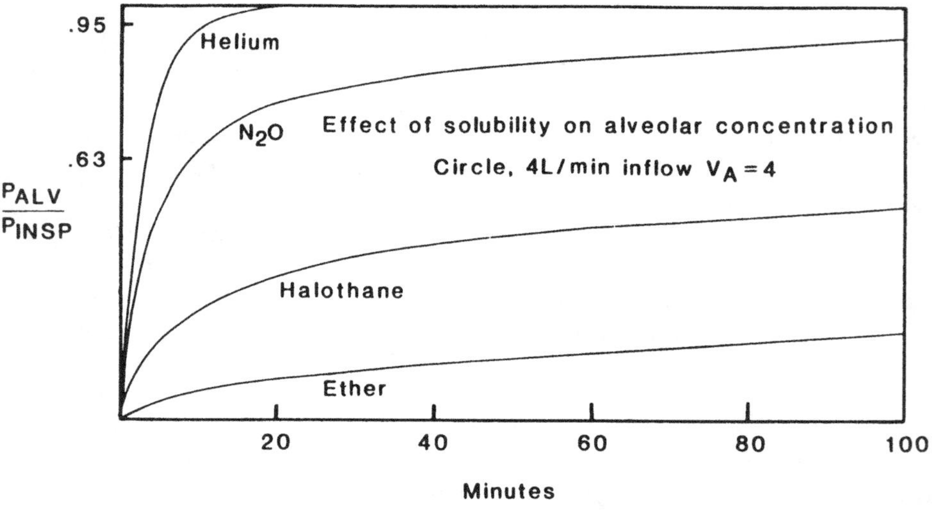

FIGURE 5.3 *Curves drawn by the electrical analog, illustrating the approach of alveolar partial pressure (P_{ALV}) to the inflowing partial pressure (P_{INSP}) in a breathing circuit with an 8-L volume of gases of varying solubility. V_A denotes alveolar ventilation. (Reproduced with permission from Severinghaus JW: Role of lung factors. In: Papper EM, Kitz JR, eds. Uptake and distribution of anesthetic agents. New York: McGraw-Hill, 1962:63.)*

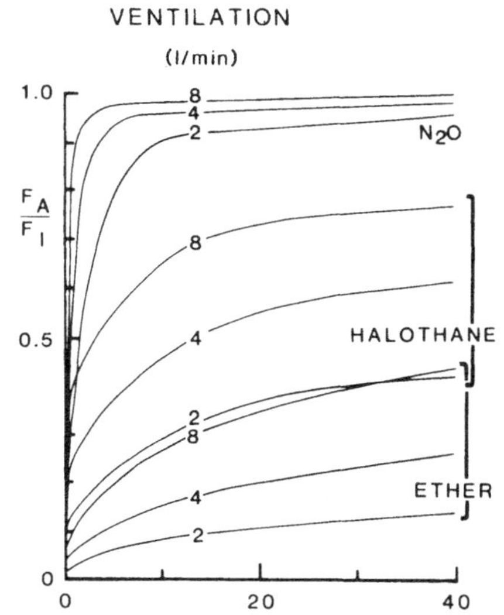

FIGURE 5.4 *The alveolar rate of rise toward the inspired concentration (F_A/F_I) is accelerated by an increase in alveolar ventilation from 2 to 4 and from 4 to 8 L/min (constant cardiac output). This effect is greater with the more soluble anesthetics than with the less soluble ones. (Reproduced with permission from Eger EI II: Anesthetic uptake and action. Baltimore: Williams and Wilkins, 1976:123.)*

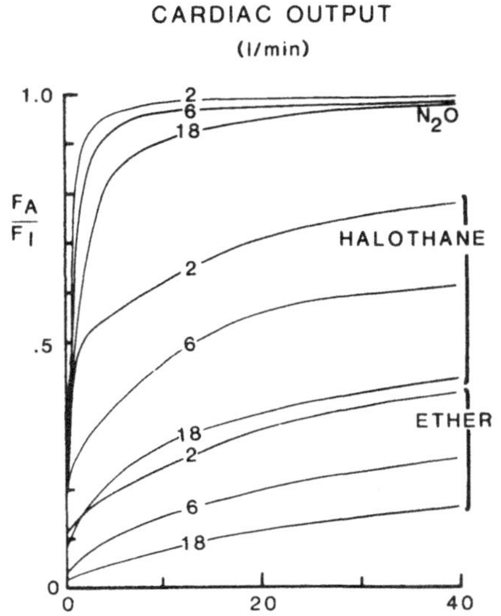

FIGURE 5.5 *If ventilation is held constant, then increases in cardiac output of from 2 to 6 to 18 L/min will increase uptake and consequently retard the rate of increase of the alveolar concentration (F_A) toward the concentration inspired (F_I). This effect is greatest with the more soluble anesthetics. These graphs presume that changes in cardiac output affect all tissues proportionately. (Reproduced with permission from Eger EI II: Anesthetic uptake and action. Baltimore: Williams and Wilkins, 1976:131.)*

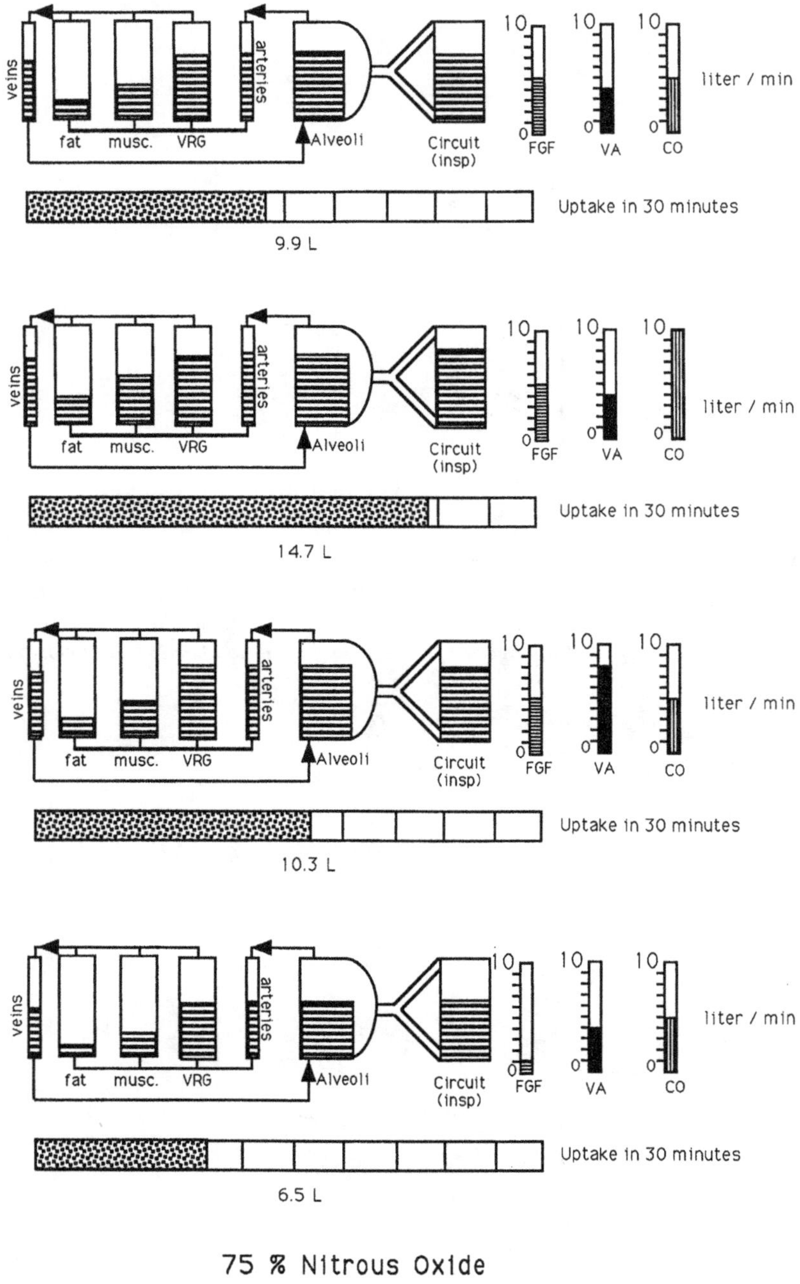

FIGURE 5.6 *Altering cardiac output (CO), alveolar ventilation (VA), or fresh gas flow (FGF) affects the distribution of anesthetic agents in the different compartments and the total amount taken up by the body. Data shown here, representing 30 minutes of nitrous oxide administration, were obtained with the Gas Man computer program. insp denotes inspired gas concentration; VRG the vessel rich group.*

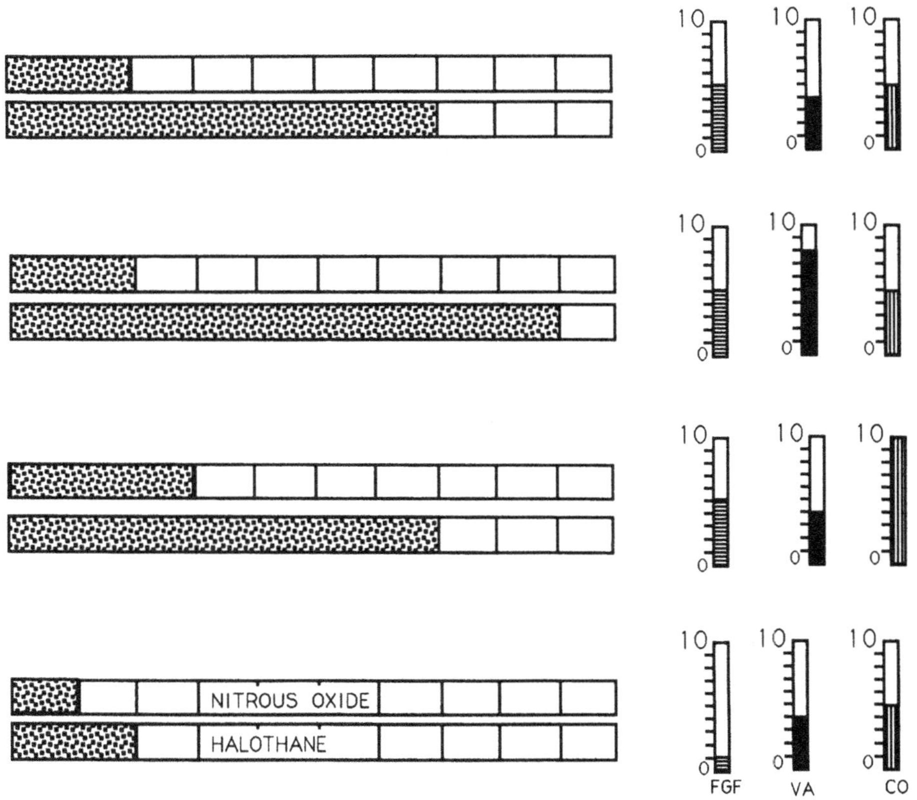

FIGURE 5.7 *Solubility affects the amount of anesthetic agent taken up by the body. After 10 minutes of administration of either 5% nitrous oxide* (upper bar) *or 5% halothane* (lower bar), *the total uptake of halothane (gas/blood solubility coefficient of 2.3) greatly exceeds that of 5% nitrous oxide (gas/blood solubility coefficient of 0.47). The data, obtained with the help of the Gas Man computer program, assume identical and steady cardiac output and ventilation for both examples.*

the flow rate of fresh gas, from 5 L/min to 1 L/min in our example, has a large effect. Doubling cardiac output causes more uptake of nitrous oxide than does doubling ventilation. Solubility has an important role in the uptake of anesthetic (Figure 5.7). While many anesthetics (and certainly 5% halothane) powerfully affect ventilation, cardiac output, and organ blood flow, in order to demonstrate the effects of solubility the data do not reflect these pharmacodynamic effects.

Unfortunately, nothing is ever straightforward. Many anesthetic agents are soluble in plastic and rubber. Therefore, some of these agents are taken up by plastic or rubber components of the anesthesia system during induction and "exhaled" by them during the patient's emergence from anesthesia. Considerable differences in solubility in plastic and rubber exist between anesthetic agents. Halothane, for example, is much more soluble than isoflurane.[3]

REFERENCES

1. Philip JH: Gas Man—an example of goal-oriented computer-assisted teaching which results in learning. Int J Clin Monit Comput 1986; 3:165–173
2. Severinghaus JW: Role of lung factors. In: Papper EM, Kitz JR, eds. Uptake and distribution of anesthetic agents. New York: McGraw-Hill, 1962:59–71
3. Targ AG, Yasuda N, Eger EI II: Solubility of I-653, sevoflurane, isoflurane, and halothane in plastics and rubber composing a conventional anesthetic circuit. Anesth Analg 1989; 69:218–225

Chapter 6

Monitoring the Function of the Anesthesia Machine, the Breathing Circuit, and the Ventilator

In modern anesthesia, the patient's airway is connected to one of a number of breathing systems that mixes and delivers physiologic and anesthetic vapors and gases. These systems carry a confusion of names; for example, several commonly used Mapleson systems are known by the names of persons who have modified or popularized them. In this text I shall use the term "Mapleson systems" generically to refer to systems that contain no carbon dioxide absorber (Figure 6.1),[1] and "circle systems" to refer to valved systems with carbon dioxide absorption.

To monitor both the inspired and end-tidal gases of a patient, it is advisable to sample them close to the patient's airway. In patients with small tidal volumes, it would be advantageous to sample the gases in the trachea or in the endotracheal tube; often, however, that is clinically not feasible, and it risks the aspiration of mucus into the sampling tube.

To monitor the functions of anesthesia machine, ventilator, and breathing circuit, we can test fresh gas before it enters the breathing circuit, and the gas in the inspiratory and expiratory hoses of the breathing circuit. Monitoring fresh gas before it enters the breathing circuit has two advantages: the gas is bone dry, and the analyzer need not have a rapid response rate, as gas concentration changes only when we adjust gas flow and vaporizer. An analyzer with a 2000-ms, 10%-to-90% rise time (see Chapter 15) could serve. But such an analyzer cannot trace the changes in gas concentration from one breath to the next or from inspiration to expiration. With a respiratory rate (RR) of only 20 breaths/min and an inspiratory-to-expiratory ratio (I:E) of 1:2, the patient spends 20 sec of every minute inhaling and 40 sec exhaling. One inspiration, therefore, occupies about 1 sec. During spontaneous ventilation, gas does not flow uniformly during that second but starts with a slow flow rate, builds up to perhaps as much as 800 ml/sec, and then slows again before exhalation starts.

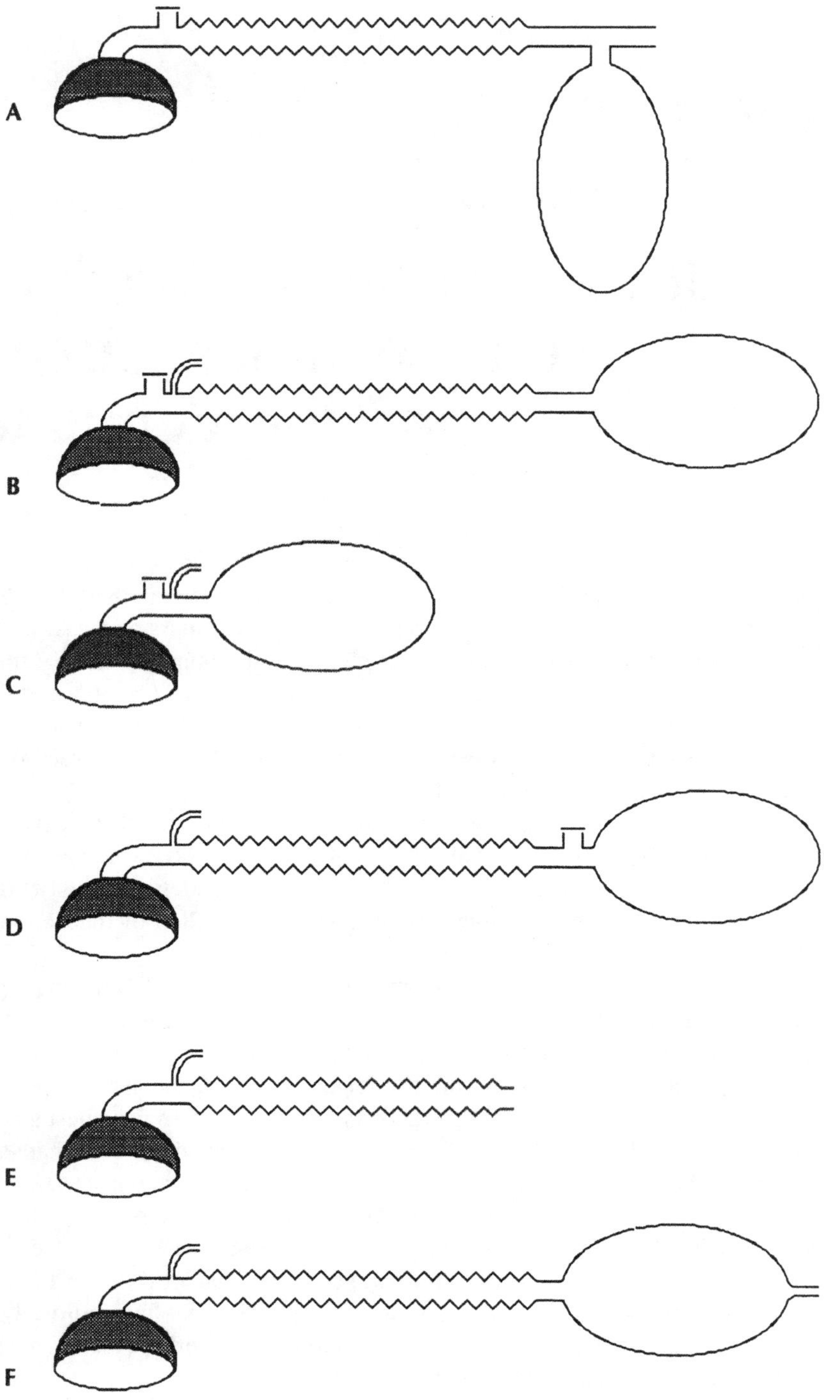
A
B
C
D
E
F

With some mechanical ventilators, the inspiratory pneumotachogram may assume the appearance of a square wave. Recording these changes of gas concentration faithfully requires a gas analyzer with a rise time less than 300 ms.[2] Monitoring gases close to the patient's trachea or endotracheal tube gives us good information about inspired gases after they have been mixed in the anesthesia breathing system, and about expired gases before they have been mixed in the breathing system. As we shall see, the site close to the mouth can provide good information on oxygen concentration in inspired gas, on valve malfunctions of circle systems, on exhausted carbon dioxide absorbers with carbon dioxide channeling through the absorber or bypassing it, and on insufficient FGF in Mapleson systems.

ANESTHESIA MACHINE WITH CIRCLE BREATHING SYSTEM

In a typical combination of anesthesia machine, ventilator, and breathing circle (Figure 6.2), together with a sidestream sampling site for respired gases, the circle system can admit fresh gas on either one side of the carbon dioxide absorber or the other—that is, between absorber and inspiratory valve (position 13a) or between absorber and expiratory valve (position 13b). Fresh gas admitted at 13b is swept with the recycled gas toward the patient during inspiration; this means the fresh gas is funneled through the carbon dioxide absorber. During expiration, the fresh gas admitted at 13a cannot reach the patient, because the inspiratory valve is closed, and the fresh gas must flow backward through the absorber.

The question arises whether fresh gas can open the inspiratory and expiratory valves during the respiratory pause and thus pass the sampling site. With the relatively low FGF in adult breathing circuits, gas follows the least resistance to flow by going directly to the ventilator and its spill valve during mechanical ventilation or, during spontaneous ventilation, to the pop-off valve (formally known as the adjustable pressure-limiting [APL] valve). With a higher FGF, some of the gas may flow through the circle. This has been described for a low-compliance, low-volume pediatric circle breathing system with flow rates as low as 4 L/min.[3]

◀ **FIGURE 6.1** *Anesthesia breathing systems, classified A through F by Mapleson. The nomenclature suggested by Mapleson has been widely adopted to describe the different arrangements of fresh gas inlet, breathing bag, and relief outlet for excess gas. (Reproduced with permission.[1]) These arrangements have been called T-piece systems or rebreathing systems.*

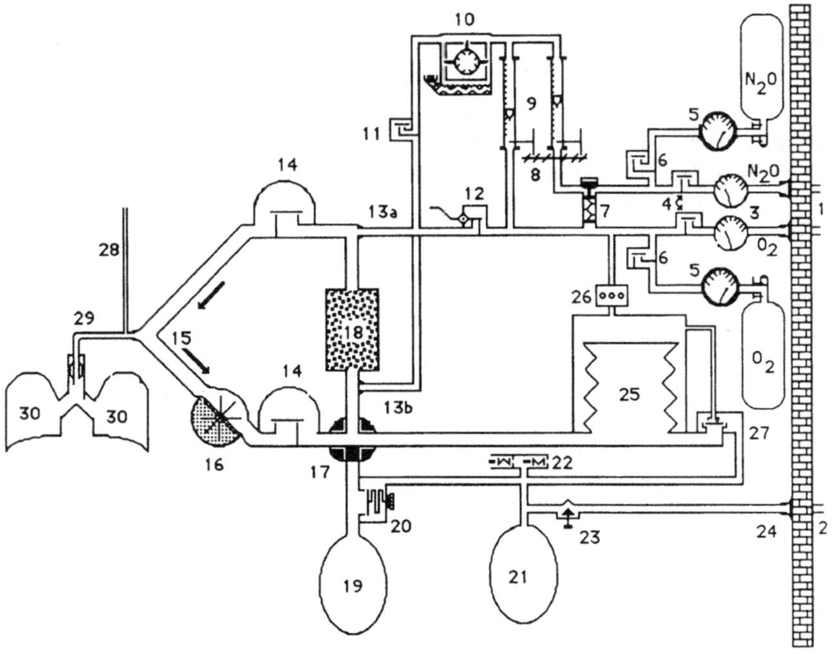

FIGURE 6.2 *A generic anesthesia machine with a circle breathing system. Details of the machine vary among manufacturers. The features of this machine are shown with easy-to-understand symbols rather than with engineering icons. The symbols represent function rather than design. Fresh gas may be admitted to the breathing circuit on either side of the carbon dioxide absorber. Where fresh gas is admitted is of little consequence clinically. However, when entering between the inspiratory valve and the absorber, fresh gas will flow during expiration (when the inspiratory valve is closed) through the absorber, toward the breathing bag or ventilator bellows. This can affect the shape of the oxygram and anesthetigram.*

Gas Supply

1. *Central gas supply*
2. *Central vacuum*
3. *Pressure gauges for piped oxygen and nitrous oxide*
4. *One-way valve: prevents loss of gas when hoses carrying piped gases are disconnected*
5. *Pressure gauges for oxygen and nitrous oxide cylinders, with pressure-regulating function*
6. *Valves preventing flow of oxygen (nitrous oxide) from cylinders, as long as pipes carrying gas from the central gas supply are connected and pressurized*
7. *Oxygen-pressure failure protection ("oxygen fail-safe"): stops nitrous oxide flow when oxygen pressure falls*
8. *Oxygen proportioning device: makes it impossible to deliver less than preset proportion of oxygen (usually 25%) in gas mixture*
9. *Flowmeter tubes and floats*
10. *Vaporizer*
11. *Device that minimizes pressure transmission from breathing circuit to vaporizer*
12. *Oxygen flush valve*
13. *Common gas outlets, (a) between inspiratory valve and absorber, (b) or, as an option, between absorber and expiratory valve*

DISCONNECTION AND LEAKS

Unrecognized disconnection of gas conduits in the anesthesia machine is among the common problems with potentially fatal consequences.[4] The minimal monitoring standards propagated by the American Society of Anesthesiologists (ASA) and the group of hospitals affiliated with Harvard Medical School[5,6] specifically address means of detecting disconnection before it alters vital signs of the patient. According to the ASA, "When ventilation is controlled by a mechanical ventilator, there shall be in continuous use a device that is capable of detecting disconnection of components of the breathing system. The device must give an audible signal when its alarm threshold is exceeded."[5] A capnograph with an apnea alarm meets this requirement.

Disconnections occur at several typical sites (Figure 6.3). Whether the ventilator's bellows rises or falls with expiration also plays a role. A ventilator with a weighted bellows that aspirates gas during expiration will continue to work even after the disconnection of gas conduits (Figure 6.4). Instead of filling with the patient's exhaled gas, the weighted bellows aspirates room air through the disconnected tubing. With the next inspiration, the air leaks out again instead of being delivered to the patient. Capnography reveals that no expired gas reaches the sampling port.

Breathing Circuit

14. *Inspiratory and expiratory valve*
15. *Y piece*
16. *Bidirectional respirometer*
17. *Selector switch*
18. *Carbon dioxide absorber*
19. *Breathing bag*
20. *Adjustable pressure-limiting (APL), or "pop-off," valve*
21. *Scavenging reservoir bag*
22. *Valve to compensate for excessive pressure or excessive suction*
23. *Control for adjusting suction*
24. *Connection to central vacuum*

Ventilator

25. *Ventilator bellows*
26. *Ventilator power supply (here, oxygen) and controls*
27. *Ventilator pressure relief valve: dumps gas from breathing circuit to scavenging system late in expiration, when bellows reaches top of box*

Gas Monitoring System

28. *Capillary, through which gas is aspirated for analysis*

Physiologic System

29. *Endotracheal tube*
30. *Lungs*

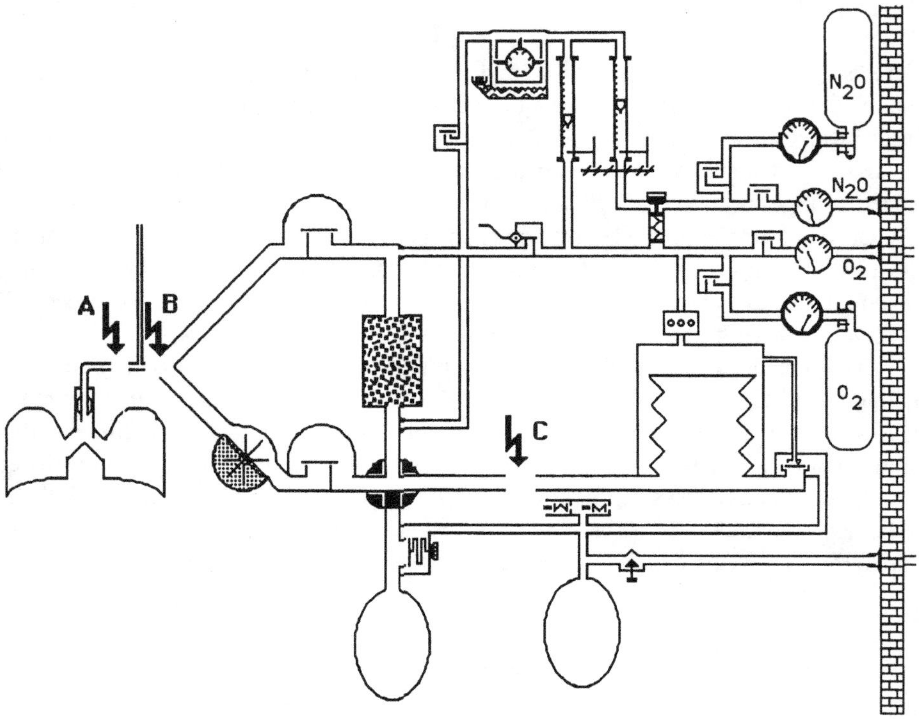

FIGURE 6.3 *In the apneic patient dependent on mechanical ventilation, a disconnection at site A, B, or C causes all respiratory fluctuations to disappear from the capnogram, the oxigram, and the anesthetigram. The tracings are arrested at their last values and then gradually reflect room air readings as air is drawn into the sampling chamber.*

In a spontaneously breathing patient, the site of disconnection is important. In the case of a disconnection at site A, the readings are the same as those for a disconnection at the same site in a patient dependent on mechanical ventilation.

With a disconnection at site B, the gas monitors show respiratory fluctuations of carbon dioxide, oxygen, and anesthetic agent. However, inspired values of anesthetic agent are zero, and oxygen values reflect room air. This is one of the few conditions in which agent monitoring helps in the differential diagnosis of a disconnection.

With a disconnection at the ventilator hose (site C), the capnogram will reflect spontaneous ventilation. However, room air will dilute the oxygen and agent concentrations, unless the fresh gas flow is so high as to prevent room air from reaching the patient during inspiration.

With a bellows that rises during expiration, a disconnection can be discovered much more readily. Normally, the patient's expired gas pushes the bellows up; this will not happen after a disconnection. But even here, it is possible for the bellows and the respirometer to deceive the clinician. In some ventilators, an empty bellows is compressed beyond its empty, resting position during mechanical inspiration. At the end

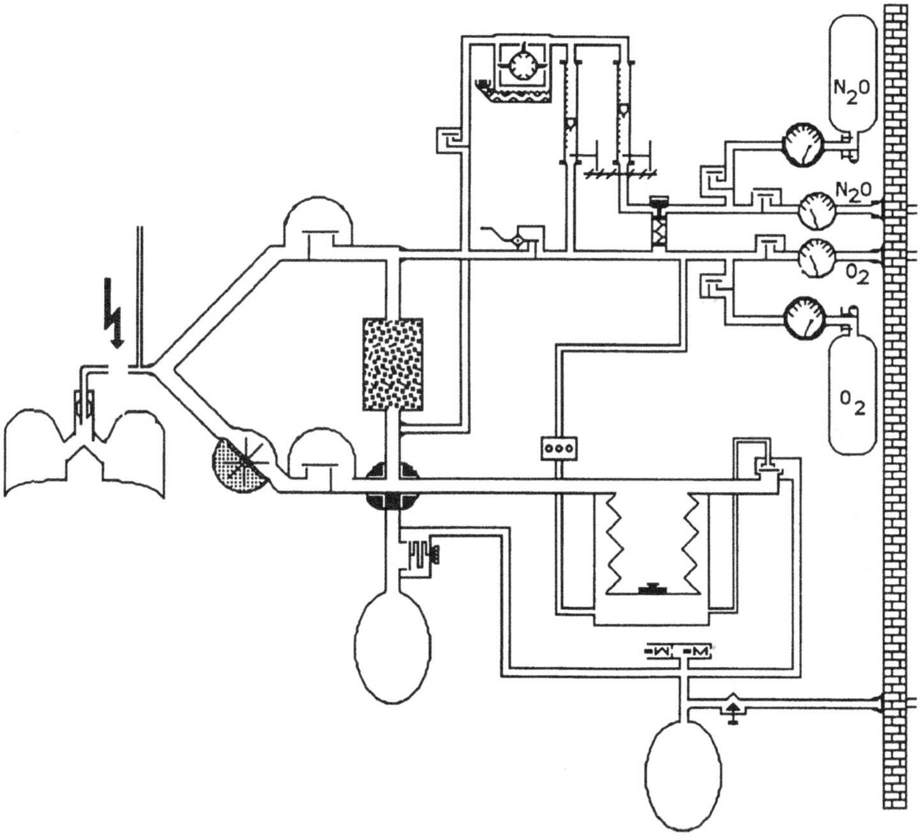

FIGURE 6.4 *If the bellows descends by gravity during exhalation in a patient undergoing mechanical ventilation, the ventilator does not cease to operate if there is a large leak or disconnection. A hanging bellows aspirates room air through the disconnection or the large leak and continues to function, even though the gas delivered by the ventilator escapes into the room during inspiration. Capnography is the best means of discovering this type of disconnection.*

of inspiration, when the ventilator rests, the compressed bellows, recoiling to its resting position, aspirates gas through the disconnection. We have seen between 50 and 150 ml of gas aspirated under different experimental conditions.[7] Again, a capnogram indicates the absence of ventilation. Either no carbon dioxide is detected in the expired gas (which was aspirated through the leak instead of from the patient), or the capnogram shows the last $P_{ET}CO_2$ value if the disconnection occurred late in expiration—for example, at site C (Figure 6.3)—but there will be no repetitive capnogram. The result is that the carbon dioxide analyzer sounds an apnea alarm.

Less obvious than a disconnection is an insidious leak that may lead to hypoventilation and hypoxemia. For instance, leaving the filler cap off the vaporizer provides

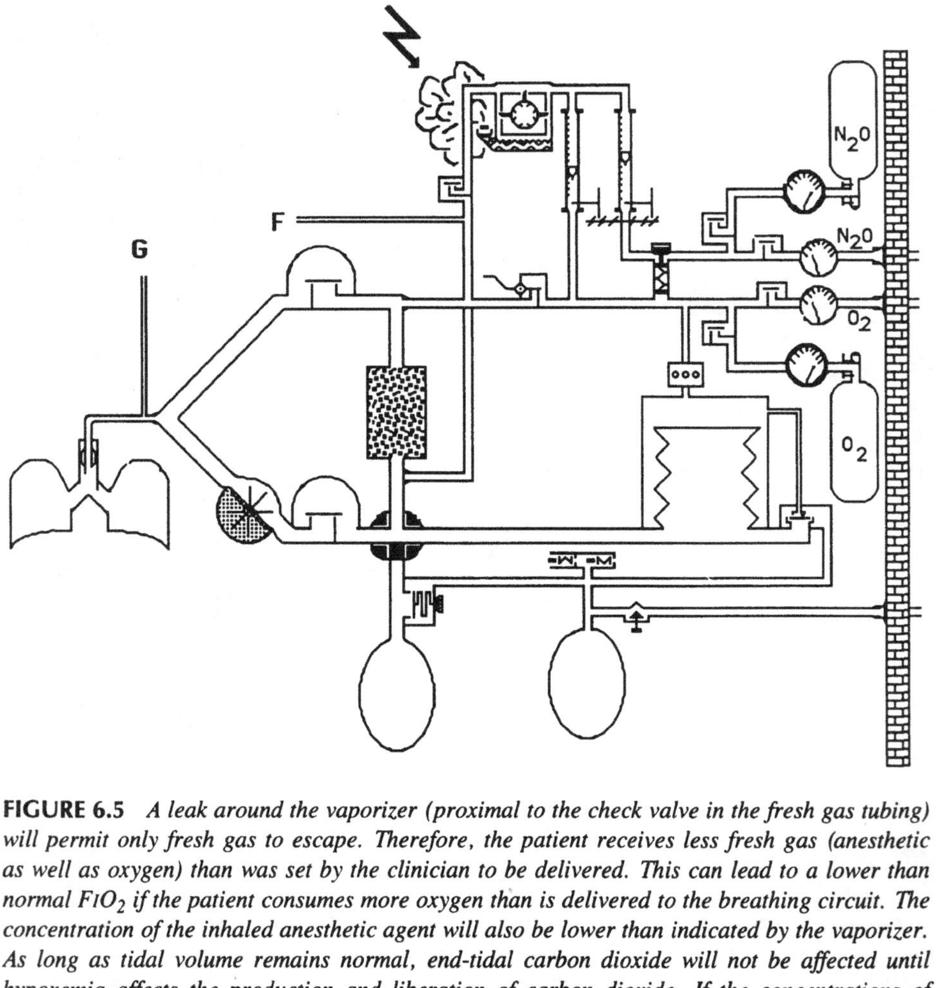

FIGURE 6.5 *A leak around the vaporizer (proximal to the check valve in the fresh gas tubing) will permit only fresh gas to escape. Therefore, the patient receives less fresh gas (anesthetic as well as oxygen) than was set by the clinician to be delivered. This can lead to a lower than normal* F_IO_2 *if the patient consumes more oxygen than is delivered to the breathing circuit. The concentration of the inhaled anesthetic agent will also be lower than indicated by the vaporizer. As long as tidal volume remains normal, end-tidal carbon dioxide will not be affected until hypoxemia affects the production and liberation of carbon dioxide. If the concentrations of oxygen and anesthetic agent are monitored in the fresh-gas tubing at site F, the problem will be difficult to diagnose. Monitoring gases at sample port G will reveal the problem.*

an escape for much fresh gas (Figure 6.5). The problem is not readily discovered if only fresh gas is analyzed (Figure 6.5, sample port F). The total volume of gas delivered to the breathing circle is reduced because of the leak. This is a dangerous problem. The ventilator can continue to work normally because enough total gas volume is delivered into the breathing circuit to satisfy ventilation in the rebreathing system. The FO_2 in this fresh gas may be well above the minimal 0.2, but an insufficient volume of oxygen in the fresh gas may not satisfy the patient's requirement for oxygen. The inspired gas mixture can grow progressively more hypoxic (Table 6.1).

Table 6.1 The Rate of Decline of FIO_2 in a Circle System with a Capacity of 5 L

	Time (Minutes)				
	1	*2*	*3*	*4*	*5*
At beginning of minute the circle breathing system starts with:					
FIO_2	0.25	0.214	0.189	0.164	0.139
N_2O	3750	3930	4055	4180	4305
O_2	1250	1070	945	820	695
Consumed during minute:					
N_2O	0	0	0	0	0
O_2	250	250	250	250	250
Added during minute:					
N_2O	375	375	375	375	375
O_2	125	125	125	125	125
After venting excess gas of 250 ml, there remains in system at end of minute:					
FIO_2	0.214	0.189	0.164	0.139	0.114

The addition of fresh gas exceeds the patient's gas consumption, yet it leads to hypoxia. All gas quantities are expressed in milliliters. Assume equilibrium with nitrous oxide and oxygen consumption of 250 ml/min, complete absorption of carbon dioxide. Respiratory quotient = 1. Fresh gas is added at a rate of 4 L/min (1 L oxygen and 3 L nitrous oxide), of which only 500 ml reaches the circle system because of a large leak around the vaporizer. See text and Figure 1.2.

Imagine that an anesthetist had elected to use 4 L/min of fresh gas. Because of the unrecognized leak, only 1.0 L/min of fresh gas (with an FO_2 of 0.25 and a flow rate of 250 ml of oxygen per minute) reached the circle system. The patient removed only 250 ml of oxygen per minute from the circle system, which had a total internal volume (ventilator bellows, tubes, carbon dioxide absorber canister) of 5 L. The ventilator breathing circuit, therefore, never ran out of gas, but the FO_2 decreased inexorably. Oxygen analysis in the inspired limb of the breathing circle or close to the patient's mouth could have detected the problem. A similar scenario was programmed into a computer-driven simulator (Figure 6.6). The ASA says, "During every administration of general anesthesia using an anesthesia machine, the concentration of oxygen in the patient breathing system shall be measured by an oxygen analyzer with a low oxygen concentration limit alarm in use."[5]

A leak can also lurk at the junction between carbon dioxide absorber and anesthesia machine, where kernels of carbon dioxide absorbent are caught at the gasket

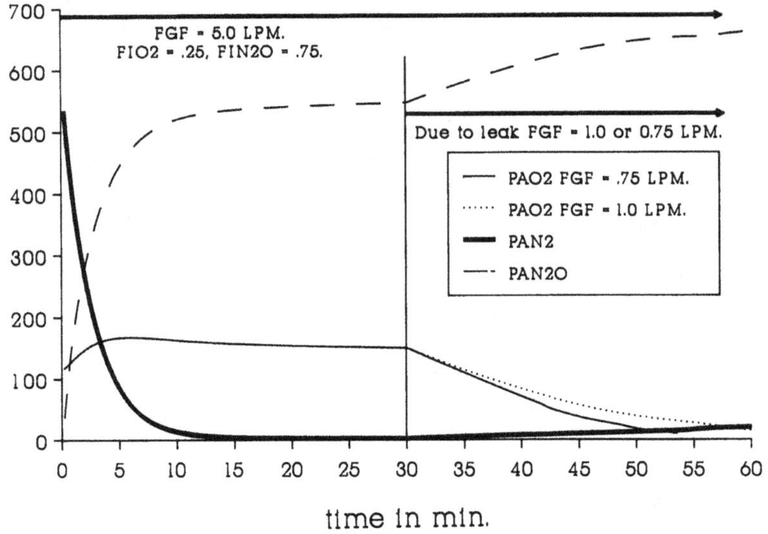

FIGURE 6.6 *Hypoxic gas mixtures are possible even though the fresh gas contains 25% oxygen. The graph is a computer-generated plot of alveolar gas concentrations (mm HG) in a patient breathing with the help of a circle system and mechanical ventilation. The patient's oxygen (O_2) consumption is set at 250 ml/min. Anesthesia with nitrous oxide (N_2O) and oxygen begins at minute 0. The fresh gas flow (FGF) into the circle system is 5 L/min. Observe the washout of nitrogen (N_2). A leak develops in the fresh gas supply at minute 30, and only 0.75 L/min or 1 L/min of the gas mixture containing 25% oxygen and 75% nitrous oxide enters the breathing circle. Observe the decreasing alveolar oxygen tension (P_AO_2) (shown for both 1 L/min and 0.75 L/min) and the increasing alveolar tension of nitrous oxide (P_AN_2O) (interrupted curve, shown for 1 L/min only). Because the patient continues to remove oxygen at a rate of 250 ml/min but removes almost no nitrous oxide, the gas in the breathing circle gradually becomes hypoxic. Observe the appearance of nitrogen in the alveoli (P_AN_2) at minute 40 and later (shown only for 1 L/min flow). The first washout of nitrogen has reduced P_AN_2 to almost zero; relatively little exhaled nitrogen was reinhaled, owing to the relatively great FGF of 5 L/min. With the low FGF of 1 L/min, some of the nitrogen being washed out of poorly perfused compartments becomes measurable. (Graph prepared by J.J. Heffels.)*

(Figure 6.7). This leak is usually easy to detect by checking the anesthesia machine before each use. Simply pressurize the breathing circuit and watch whether the system holds the pressure. A sizable leak at this junction will also lead to hypoventilation. Yet more gas will be lost from the leak close to the vaporizer than from the one close to the carbon dioxide absorber, even if the leaks are of the same size (say, 3 mm in diameter), because the gas pressure in the tubing that connects the vaporizer is higher than the pressure around the carbon dioxide absorber, which never exceeds peak inspiratory pressure during mechanical ventilation.

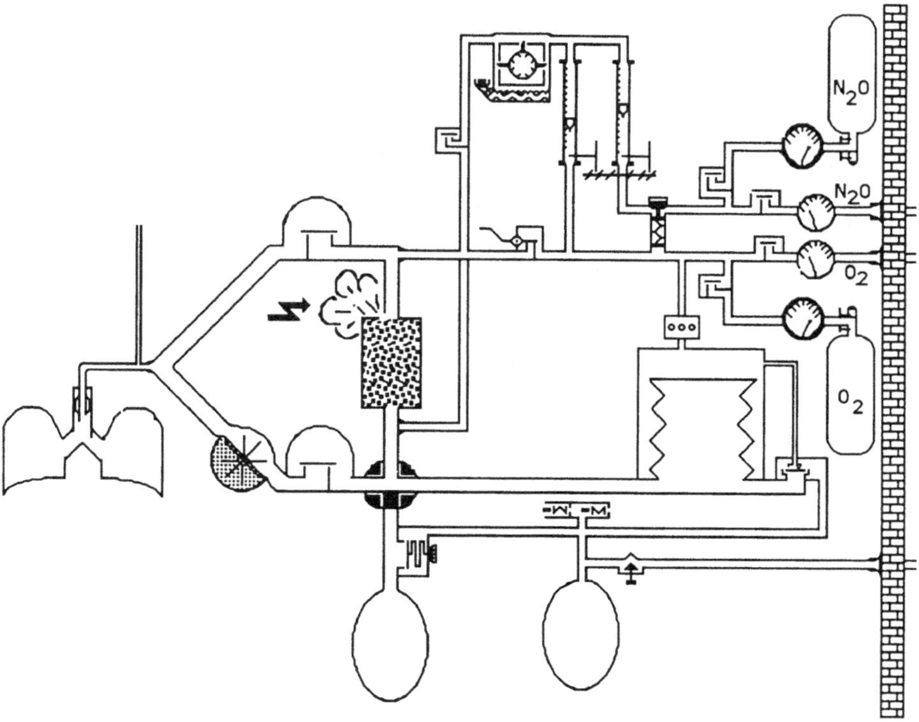

FIGURE 6.7 *With a leak separated from the patient by two competent valves (for instance, around the carbon dioxide absorber), a part of the tidal volume delivered by the ventilator is lost to the outside. The patient becomes hypoventilated, and end-tidal carbon dioxide increases while inspired oxygen decreases. Anesthetic agents change correspondingly.*

It is important to test not only the breathing circuit for leaks (easily done) but also the machine itself. The latter requires more effort. Vaporizers must be tested individually and according to the instructions of the machine's manufacturer. In some machines, testing for leaks calls for disconnecting all pipelines and closing the cylinders, opening all flowmeters, and applying a suction bulb to the common gas outlet to determine whether the mild vacuum of the suction bulb is maintained for 30 sec.

A leak between the patient's mouth or endotracheal tube and the one-way valves in the breathing circuit generates a specific type of capnogram. A leak close to the inspiratory valve will cause fresh gas to be lost during mechanical inspiration, which reduces the patient's tidal volume and thus leads to hypoventilation and increased P_{ETCO_2}. If the leak is large enough to accommodate escaping gas during expiration, end-tidal gas containing carbon dioxide will reach the inspiratory limb. During the next inspiration, this gas will be pushed back and past the gas-sampling port. A capnogram with a sloped phase IV typically results (Figure 6.8a). Capnographically, this is

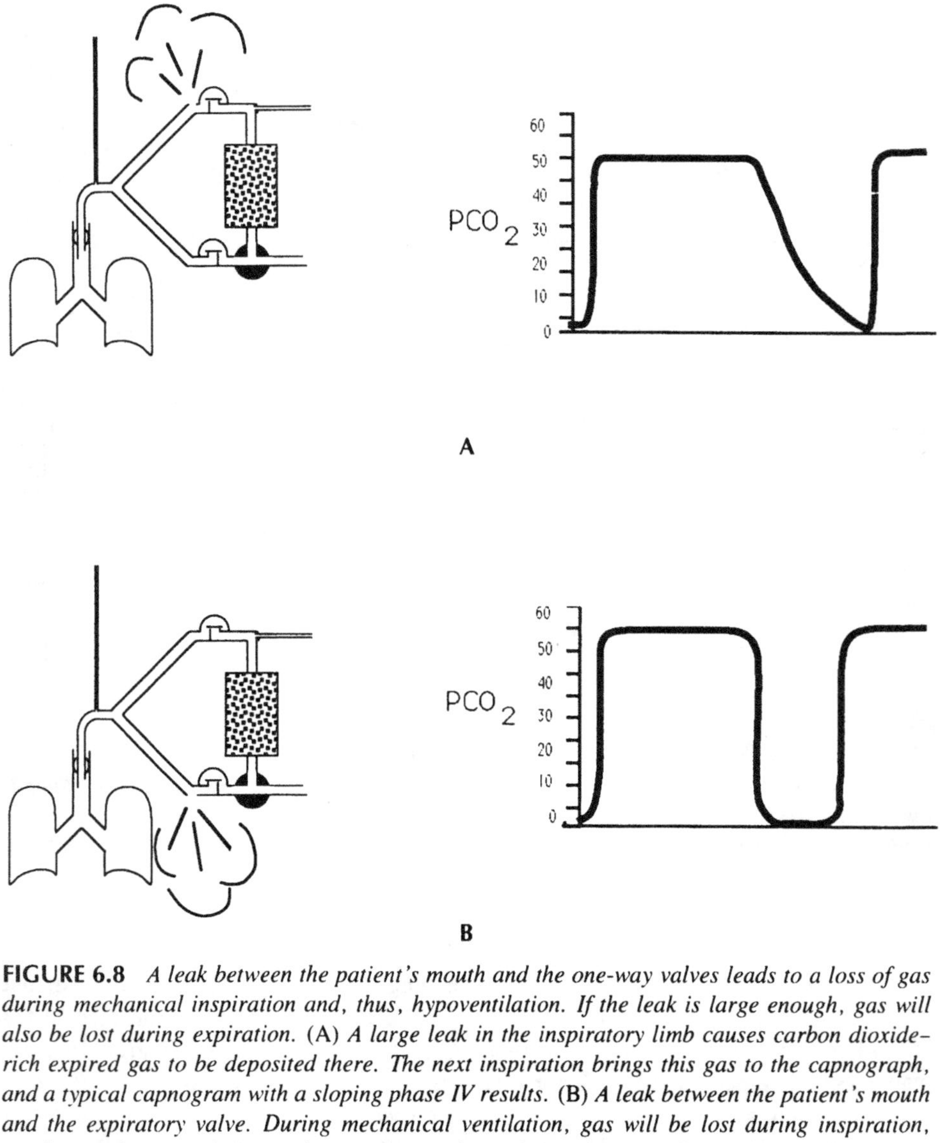

FIGURE 6.8 *A leak between the patient's mouth and the one-way valves leads to a loss of gas during mechanical inspiration and, thus, hypoventilation. If the leak is large enough, gas will also be lost during expiration.* (A) *A large leak in the inspiratory limb causes carbon dioxide–rich expired gas to be deposited there. The next inspiration brings this gas to the capnograph, and a typical capnogram with a sloping phase IV results.* (B) *A leak between the patient's mouth and the expiratory valve. During mechanical ventilation, gas will be lost during inspiration, resulting in hypoventilation and a capnogram that indicates hypoventilation (high end-tidal carbon dioxide) but normal configuration.*

indistinguishable from an incompetent inspiratory valve (see below). If the leak is close to the expiratory valve but between the valve and the patient's mouth, and if enough gas is spilled (Figure 6.8b), the capnogram shows evidence of hypoventilation. No evidence of such a leak is apparent on the capnogram during mechanical inspiration.

MALFUNCTION OF VALVES AND CARBON DIOXIDE ABSORBER

Capnography can also indicate whether the carbon dioxide absorber and one-way valves work properly. When carbon dioxide appears in inspired gas, we have evidence of rebreathing; either the gas was not scrubbed by the absorber (because of an exhausted absorber, channeling through absorber kernels that are too loosely packed, or because of an open bypass valve) or one or both one-way valves are malfunctioning.

Valves fail, for example, when the expiratory valve becomes moist and sticks in the open position, or when the valve leaflet provided by the manufacturer is replaced by a homemade surrogate cut out of a piece of radiograph film. The film warps and the valve no longer closes properly. On the capnogram, incompetence of the expiratory valve looks quite different from incompetence of the inspiratory valve. Malfunction of the inspiratory valve generates subtle changes in the capnogram. During expiration, some exhaled gas is deposited in the inspiratory limb and sits there until the next inspiration. The first part of the inspired volume, therefore, contains the carbon dioxide that was left behind in the inspiratory limb. Consequently, phase IV of the capnogram (the downstroke) cannot fall to zero as rapidly as normal, and the slope is prolonged; it may eventually return to baseline if the tidal volume is sufficiently large (Figure 6.9A). Imagine that the capnogram is examined simply for the return to baseline rather than also for the slope of phase IV. Just because phase I eventually reaches zero does not mean that there is no rebreathing. That the patient rebreathes when the slope of phase IV is slanted becomes apparent when P_{ETCO_2} slowly increases.

With malfunction of the expiratory valve, the inspiration contains the end-tidal gas that had been deposited in the expiratory hose during the previous breath. The capnogram shows an elevated phase I, indicative of increased equipment dead space. Rebreathing of carbon dioxide will reduce elimination of the gas, and the end-tidal value will increase (Figure 6.9B).

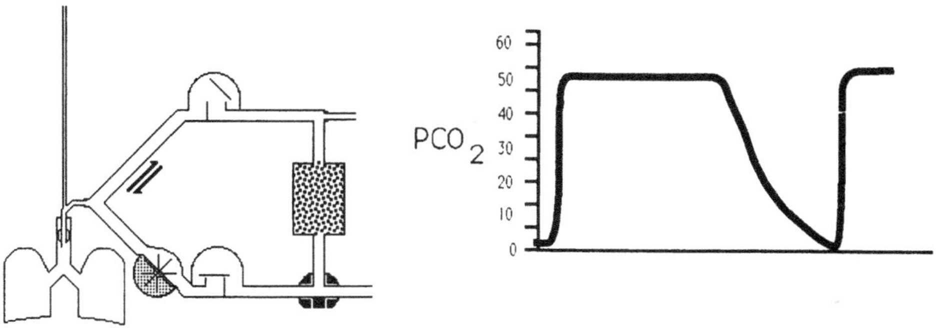

A

FIGURE 6.9(A) *Incompetent inspiratory valve results in bidirectional gas flow in the inspiratory limb of the breathing circuit. The capnogram shows characteristic slanted phase IV. The expired tidal volume indicated by the spirometer will be reduced by the amount of gas that flows back into the inspiratory limb of the breathing circuit.*

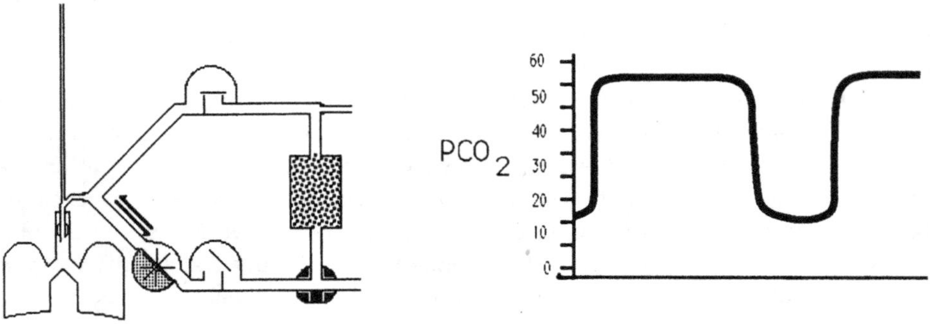

B

FIGURE 6.9(B) *Incompetent expiratory valve results in bidirectional gas flow in the expiratory limb of the breathing circuit. The capnogram shows inspired and increased end-tidal carbon dioxide (PCO_2). A spirometer reflects bidirectional flow (as shown).*

WRONG GAS

No anesthetist can trust the anesthesia system blindly. Sometimes, unbeknownst to the clinical team, the pipes carrying medicinal gases to the operating room are connected incorrectly, and a gas other than oxygen comes out of the central gas supply clearly marked "oxygen" (Figures 6.10 and 6.11, A and B). On one occasion, a faulty connection in an operating room caused nitrous oxide to flow from an anesthesia machine into the oxygen pipeline in the wall. In the neighboring operating rooms, nitrous oxide instead of oxygen was delivered from the oxygen wall outlet. Three patients died. At another institution, construction workers had inadvertently switched the oxygen and nitrous oxide pipes. As long as both flowmeters for oxygen (carrying nitrous oxide) and nitrous oxide (carrying oxygen) were in use, the patient did well. But at the end of anesthesia, the "nitrous oxide" was turned off and the patient was given pure "oxygen." She turned quite blue and eventually died because the anesthetist did not believe that anything but oxygen could come out of the oxygen flowmeter. Oxygen analysis of the inspired gas would have revealed the problem and saved the patient's life. Oxygen analyzers are not expensive. Gases must be monitored before they reach the patient! Mix-ups of pipelines are rare, but they do occur.

Oxygen analyzers in the breathing system have become a minimal standard of care in the United States. The monitor should have an adjustable alarm for both low and high oxygen concentrations, and the low levels should be set no lower than 21% (usually higher—see page 81). High alarms are needed in two circumstances:

1. While anesthetizing a premature infant, a clinician might elect to limit the FIO_2 to 40% or less (monitor PaO_2 and SpO_2) in order to minimize the chance of retrolental fibroplasia (now often called retinopathy of prematurity).

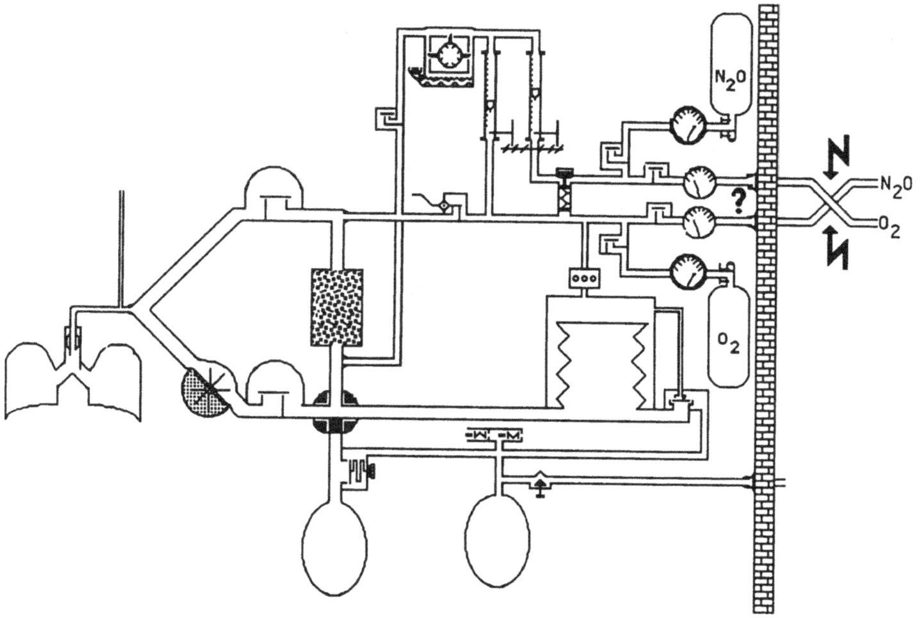

FIGURE 6.10 *Many anesthesia-related deaths have been attributed to the problem depicted here: during repairs or construction, oxygen and nitrous oxide pipes are crossed. The nitrous oxide outlet in the operating room delivers oxygen, and vice versa. As long as a 50/50 mixture of the two gases is used, the problem goes undetected. However, as soon as 100% oxygen is selected, the oxygen analyzer reports that no oxygen is detected.*

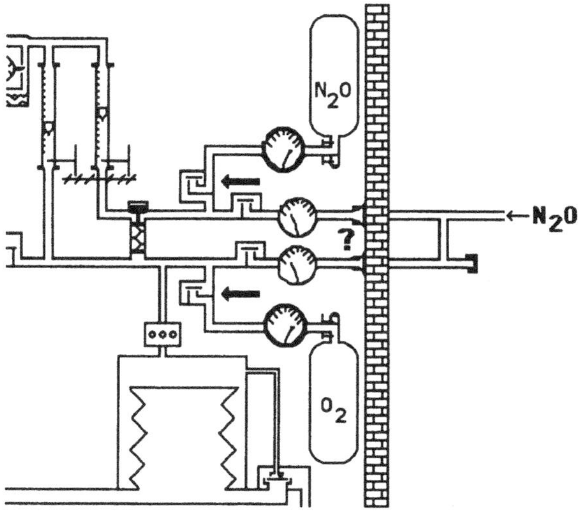

FIGURE 6.11(A) *American anesthesia machines differ from some made in other countries. In the United States, check-valves (see arrows) prevent gas in the cylinders from exiting as long as there is pressure in the central gas supply hoses, because the piped pressure exceeds the reduced pressure from the cylinders. Therefore, one must disconnect the gas supply hoses from the wall before the gas in the reserve cylinders can be used.*

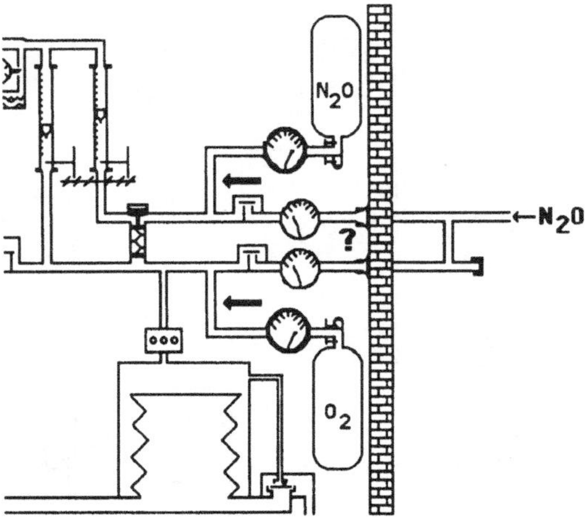

B

FIGURE 6.11(B) *With this arrangement (not typical for US anesthesia machines) the gas supply hoses do not have to be disconnected from the wall in order to use gas from the cylinders; the drawback is that oxygen may exit from the reserve cylinder even while oxygen from the central supply system is being used. Thus, the reserve cylinder may be empty when an emergency arises.*

2. Endotracheal papillomas can be vaporized and thus removed by a laser beam directed past the endotracheal tube. In one technique, a mixture of no more than 30% oxygen in helium is used as the carrier gas for the inhalation anesthetic.[8,9] This is because 70% or more helium significantly reduces the hazard of ignition of polyvinylchloride tracheal tubes when a carbon dioxide laser with an 8-mm spot size is used at 10 watts or less for 10 sec or less.

MAPLESON BREATHING SYSTEMS

So far we have discussed the circle systems in common use in many parts of the world. Anesthesia systems that funnel respired gases back and forth in separate conduits with the help of valves make capnography easy because they separate inspired gas from expired gas. Systems that rely on the clever arrangement of gas flows and spillage of excess gas to dump carbon dioxide make the interpretation of capnograms more difficult. These systems require no carbon dioxide absorber.[9] Particularly well liked are the Jackson-Rees, Bain, Lack, and Magill systems (Figure 6.12).

The Jackson-Rees System

The Jackson-Rees system requires an FGF about twice the minute volume, as long as ventilation assumes a sinusoidal pattern. When the expiratory pause is shortened, there is less time for carbon dioxide to wash out, and rebreathing is likely unless FGF exceeds twice the minute volume.

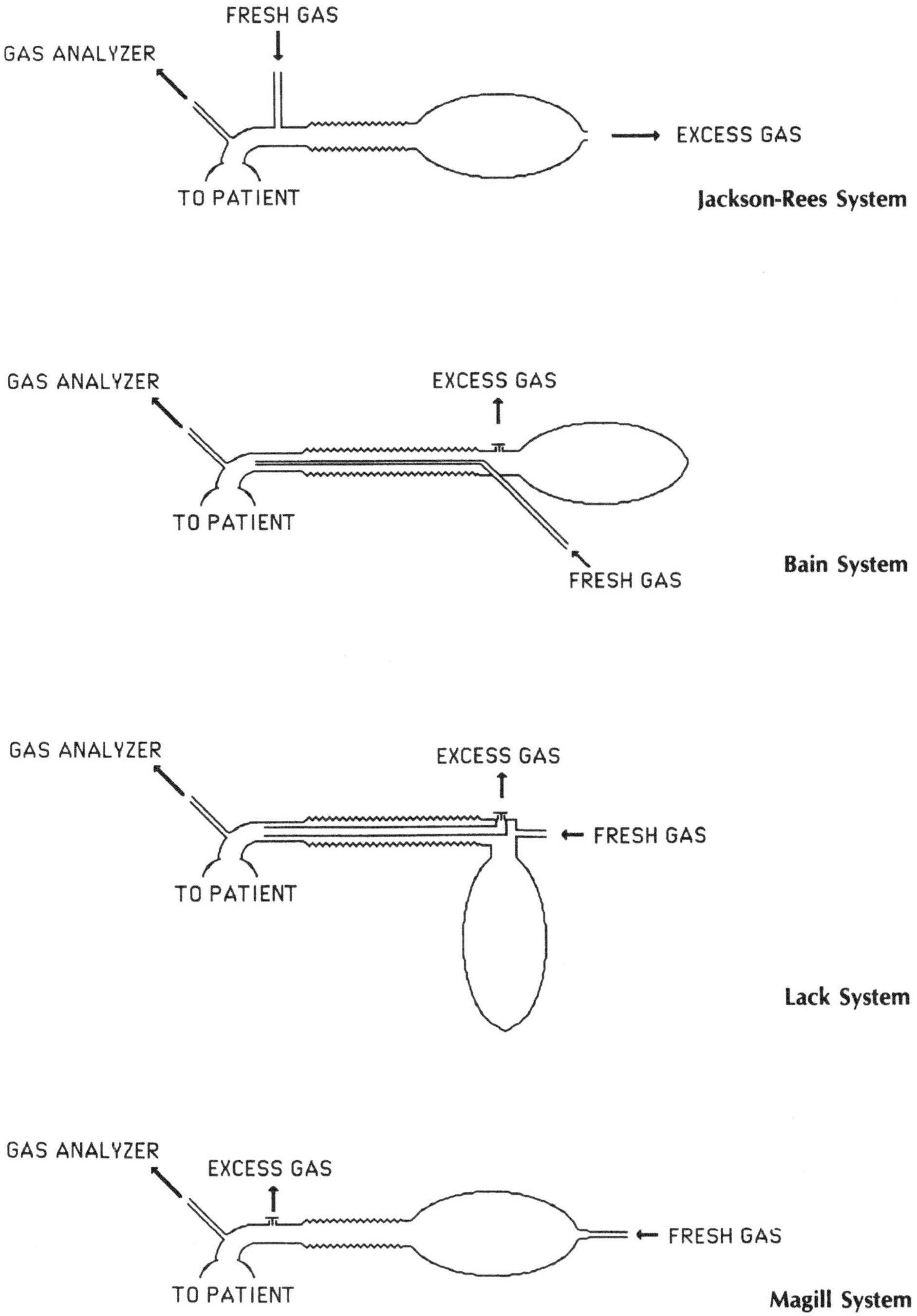

FIGURE 6.12 *Frequently used Mapleson systems known by their eponyms. The Jackson-Rees is a Mapleson F system, the Bain a modified Mapleson D system, the Lack a modified Mapleson F, and the Magill a Mapleson A.*

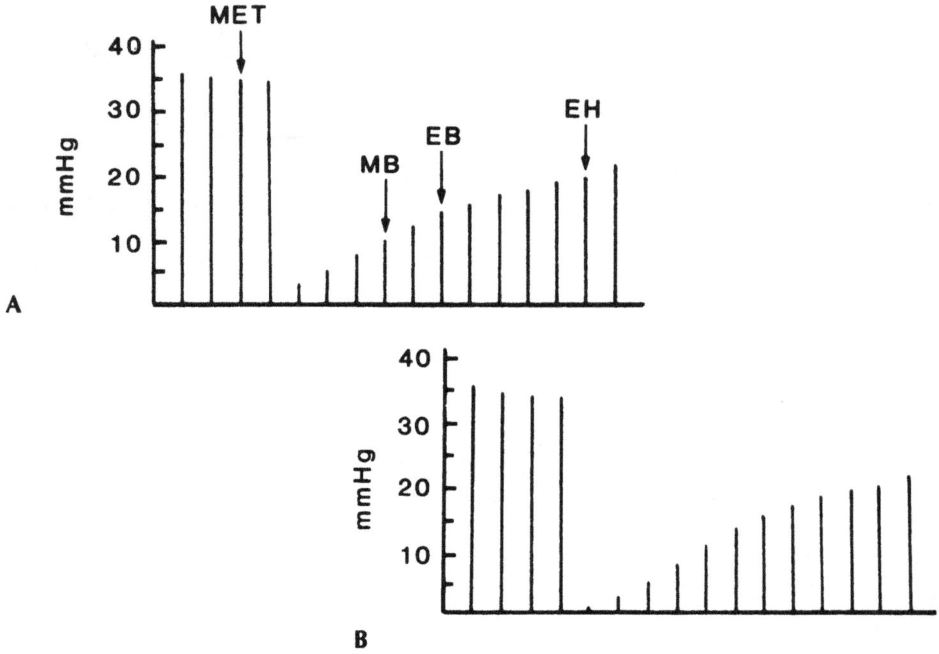

FIGURE 6.13 *Longitudinal presentation of partial pressures of carbon dioxide (PCO_2) in the Bain circuit at end-expiration, calculated by a computer model at fresh gas flow rates of 10.2 L/min* (A) *and 12.2 L/min* (B). *MET denotes midendotracheal tube; MB, middle of Bain tube; EB, end of Bain tube; EH, end of ventilator hose close to ventilator. The height of each vertical bar represents the PCO_2 in a specific segment; multiplication by the respective segmented volume yields the actual volume of carbon dioxide stored in each of the segments. The first bar on the left represents PCO_2 in the alveoli; the next three bars represent PCO_2 in three segments of the endotracheal tube. Thus, the height of the third bar from the left equals end-tidal PCO_2. The shortest bar in the graph represents the PCO_2 in the right-angle elbow connector, the next two bars that in the Bain tube and that in the hose that connects the Bain circuit with the ventilator, respectively. (Reproduced with permission.[11])*

The Bain System

The Bain system also allows fresh gas to enter close to the patient. The exhaled gas leaves the Bain system at a pop-off valve away from the patient (Figure 6.12).

The Bain system delivers fresh gas through a tube placed inside the expiratory hose.[10,11] Late in expiration, when expired gas flows slowly and then stops, the continuous flow of fresh gas washes the expired gas (rich in carbon dioxide) into the expiratory hose. With the next inspiration, fresh gas is inhaled, usually together with some of the fresh gas deposited in the expiratory hose, as well as some of the last exhaled carbon dioxide, which has been well diluted by the fresh gas. When the FGF is high enough—for example, in excess of 150 ml/kg/min—the patient should not rebreathe carbon dioxide, or at least not much.

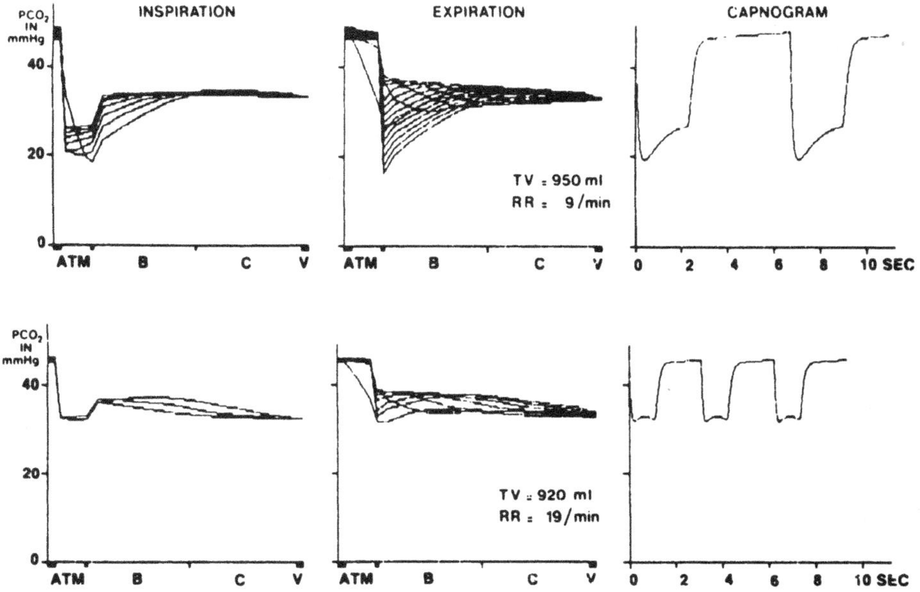

FIGURE 6.14 *Longitudinal carbon dioxide distributions (the four graphs on the left) and capnograms (the two graphs on the right) obtained from a computer model that simulates mechanical ventilation in an adult patient with a Bain system. For the longitudinal displays, the horizontal axis is a linear volume axis. Sections T, B, and C represent, respectively, volume of the anatomical dead space and endotracheal tube (in this case, 190 ml), volume of the outer volume of the Bain circuit (510 ml), and volume of the connecting tube between the ventilator and the Bain arm (558 ml). Sections A, M, and V represent, respectively, the alveolar space, the mixing area where the fresh gas enters and is mixed with the inspiratory or expiratory gas, and the ventilator. These sections are not to scale; the ordinate values at these points represent the values for partial pressure of carbon dioxide (PCO_2) in the respective volumes. Fresh gas flow rate was set at 5.2 L/min; expiratory-to-inspiratory ratio was set at 2:1; tidal volume (TV) and respiratory rate (RR) are indicated. (Reproduced with permission.[12])*

A number of variables in addition to FGF influence the propensity for rebreathing.[12] In general, the longer the expiratory pause is and the higher the FGF, the less likely is rebreathing. Considering the concentration of carbon dioxide in the trachea, the right-angle connector between endotracheal tube and Bain tube, the expiratory hose of the Bain tube, and the ventilator (Figure 6.13), it is easy to see why a lower FGF results in more rebreathing of carbon dioxide. When the clinician is using a Bain system and discovers excessive carbon dioxide in the inspired gas, the intuitive response might be to increase respiratory rate in order to increase alveolar ventilation. But this maneuver accomplishes little with the Bain system. Almost doubling minute ventilation by increasing respiratory rate has an insignificant effect on $P_{ET}CO_2$, while inspired tension actually increases further with rapid breathing (Figure 6.14).

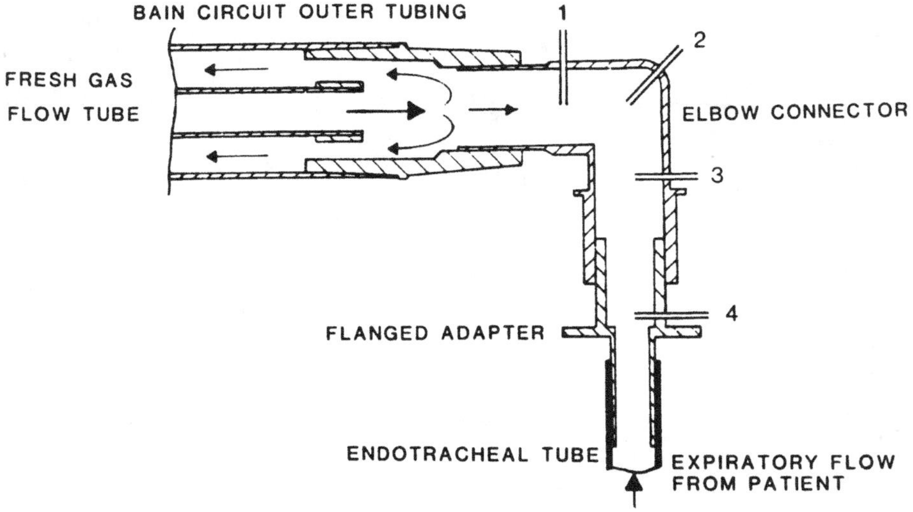

FIGURE 6.15 *Schematic of distal portion of the Bain circuit, plus connector and adapter. Sites 3 and 4 are preferable to sites 1 and 2 for sampling gas for analysis. (Reproduced with permission.[13])*

Enlarging dead space invites rebreathing. This affects not only carbon dioxide but the other gases as well. A sufficiently high FGF reduces, or even prevents, rebreathing. Most clinicians use formulas to decide how much fresh gas to use, but these formulas make a number of assumptions that may not hold for every patient. If one can measure the concentrations in inspired and expired gases, one can titrate the FGF until rebreathing is acceptable—that is, until $P_{ET}CO_2$ is normal.

The Bain system carries fresh gas close to the endotracheal tube. Sampling from within an endotracheal tube guarantees gas samples uncontaminated by fresh gas, but sampling from a pediatric endotracheal tube, for example, is clinically difficult or impossible. Sampling gases at certain sites outside the endotracheal tube yields better results than sampling at others (Figure 6.15).[13]

The Lack System

With this system, the principle of coaxial tubing was applied to a system that resembles the Magill system. The inner tubing carries the expired gas to a pressure-relief valve. If the tubes are large enough in diameter, the system works well.

The Magill System

In the Magill system, fresh gas enters at the back of the breathing bag, and the exhaust pop-off valve is positioned close to the patient. During spontaneous ventilation, this favors the venting of carbon dioxide late in expiration, when alveolar gas rich in carbon dioxide fills the trachea, the mouth, and the space around the patient's mouth. Differences in respiratory pattern influence the Magill system less than they do the Jackson-Rees system. However, the Magill system requires a higher FGF in manual ventilation to prevent rebreathing, because gas in this state is vented during inspiration when pressure in the system reaches its peak. Thus much fresh gas is lost, and gas containing carbon dioxide can reach the breathing bag unless the FGF is increased.

Even though Mapleson systems are simpler in construction than circle systems, inadequate oxygen supply in Mapleson systems is as potentially serious as it is in circle systems. Monitoring oxygen in inspired gas, therefore, remains an essential requisite for safe anesthesia. Because Mapleson systems lack carbon dioxide absorption, monitoring carbon dioxide concentration in inspired as well as end-tidal gases can assure the clinician that FGF is not so low as to cause an unacceptable level of rebreathing or so high as to be wasteful. In all Mapleson systems, FGF is often set to no less than the patient's alveolar ventilation. However, a substantially higher flow is sometimes required when a patient's pattern of breathing favors retention of carbon dioxide.[14] Different systems also behave differently with mechanical, spontaneous, or manual ventilation. With manual ventilation, excess gas escapes late during inspiration, when the pressure reaches its peak, while with spontaneous ventilation, the peak pressure causes the excess gas to be exhausted late in expiration. With mechanical ventilation, gas spillage also occurs at the end of expiration. Monitoring P_{ETCO_2} helps in selecting the appropriate FGF.

REFERENCES

1. Mapleson WW: The elimination of rebreathing in various semi-closed anaesthetic systems. Br J Anaesthesia 1954; 26:323–332
2. Selby DG, Isley AH, Runciman WB: An evaluation of five carbon dioxide analysers for use in the operating theatre and intensive care unit. Anaesth Intens Care 1987; 15:212–216
3. Schieber RA, Namnoum A, Sugden A, Saville AL, Orr RA: Accuracy of expiratory carbon dioxide measurement using the coaxial and circle breathing circuits in small subjects. J Clin Monitoring 1985; 1:149–155
4. Cooper JB, Newbower RS, Kitz RJ: An analysis of major errors and equipment failures in anesthesia management: Considerations for prevention and detection. Anesthesiology 1984; 60:34–42
5. Pierce EC Jr: Improving anesthesia safety today and in the future: Steps taken by the profession to reduce risks. In: Gravenstein JS, Holzer JF, eds. Safety and cost containment in anesthesia. Stoneham, MA: Butterworths, 1988: 105–118
6. Eichhorn JH, Cooper JB, Cullen DJ: Standards for patient monitoring during anesthesia at Harvard medical school. JAMA 1986; 256:1017–1020
7. Gravenstein JS, Nederstigt J: Monitoring for disconnection: Ventilators with bellows rising on expiration can deliver tidal volumes after disconnection. J Clin Monit, in press
8. Pashayan AG, Gravenstein JS: Helium retards endotracheal tube fires from carbon dioxide lasers. Anesthesiology 1985; 62:274–277
9. Pashayan AG, Gravenstein JS, Cassisi NJ, McLaughlin G: The helium protocol for laryngotracheal operations with carbon dioxide laser: A retrospective review of 523 cases. Anesthesiology 1988; 68:801–804

10. Conway CM: Anaesthetic breathing systems. Br J Anaesth 1985; 57:649–657
11. Beneken JEW, Gravenstein N, Gravenstein JS, van der Aa JJ, Lampotang S: Capnography and the Bain circuit I: A computer model. J Clin Monit 1985; 1:103–113
12. Beneken JEW, Gravenstein N, Lampotang S, van der Aa JJ, Gravenstein JS: Capnography and the Bain circuit II: Validation of a computer model. J Clin Monit 1987; 3:165–177
13. Gravenstein N, Lampotang S, Beneken JEW: Factors influencing capnography in the Bain circuit. J Clin Monit 1985; 1:6–10
14. Chan ASH, Bruce WE, Son N: A comparison of anaesthetic breathing systems during spontaneous ventilation. Anaesthesia 1989; 44:194–199

Chapter 7

Titration of Depth of Anesthesia

If it were possible, the anesthetist would give just enough anesthetic to abolish pain and obliterate memory. But how does one judge what is "just enough"? Clinical skill—and, often enough, a sixth sense—guide the clinician in this difficult task. Gas monitoring offers much help because it enables the clinician to assess the concentration of anesthetic agents in inspired and end-tidal gas. Before discussing this, a word about alternative methods for measuring depth of anesthesia.

The function of the central nervous system (CNS) can be monitored by recording the EEG, which works best with the help of a dozen or more leads. The limitations of the EEG include its demand for much time and attention to detail from the anesthetist, who has neither to spare, and its insensitivity once anesthesia is deep (a flat EEG means that the patient is either well anesthetized or brain-dead). Especially with light anesthesia it may be difficult to decide whether enough anesthesia has been administered to guarantee that the patient will not recall snippets of conversation made during the operation or remember having felt the surgeon's knife.

A refined method of electronic monitoring of CNS function uses evoked potentials (EPs) of the brain or spinal cord. These are the measured responses to repeated stimulation of sensory nerves in the periphery by electricity, sound, or light. With the use of sophisticated signal averaging, EPs can be detected in the background of the EEG. With deepening anesthesia, these stimuli may reach the CNS later. This method requires complex equipment and, at least at present, a specialist for EP interpretation.

EEGs and EPs are used in some centers that perform special procedures, such as carotid endarterectomy and operations on the spinal cord and aorta. At this time, neither method is recommended for routine monitoring of depth of anesthesia.

Depth of anesthesia also can be assessed by monitoring arterial BP and heart rate, because it is assumed that pain or awareness elicits sympathetic activity that raises arterial BP and heart rate. Unfortunately, BP and heart rate often rise and fall for reasons unrelated to depth of anesthesia. Conversely, hypotension is the hallmark of deep levels of inhalation anesthesia, but many other causes also lead to arterial hypotension.

MONITORING ANESTHETICS IN RESPIRED GAS

In the last few decades, it has become quite feasible clinically to monitor the concentration of inhalation anesthetics in inspired and end-tidal gas. Good information about the concentration of inhalation anesthetics required for general anesthesia is available. For inhalation agents, the minimal concentration of anesthetic agent in the alveoli (MAC) that will abolish muscular reactions to a skin incision in half of all patients ranges from 0.16 to 105 volume percent (Table 7.1).[1] MAC decreases with advancing age, with the presence of other anesthetics, with cooling, and with some medications that inhibit sympathetic function.[2] Ample evidence shows that 1.3 MAC abolishes the sensation of pain in more than 90% of all patients. Knowing the concentration of anesthetic in alveolar gas, therefore, can guide the clinician who wishes to adjust depth of anesthesia to abolish pain and produce amnesia.

Ideally we would like to know the concentration of anesthetic in brain tissue. During induction of anesthesia, the anesthetic partial pressures are highest in the circuit, lower in the alveolar gas and arterial blood, and lowest in the fat compartment. During emergence from anesthesia the concentration gradient must reverse itself.

During induction (Figure 7.1) it is often helpful to administer concentrations in the inspired gas that are much higher than needed to maintain anesthesia. These higher concentrations shorten the time of induction. This can be done safely as long as the clinician can monitor end-tidal values, which reflect arterial concentrations. During maintenance (Figure 7.2) alveolar, tissue, and venous anesthetic concentrations sooner (with less soluble agents) or later (with more soluble agents) reach equilibrium, and end-tidal gas pressures correctly reflect partial pressure of the anesthetic in brain and heart. During emergence (Figure 7.2), end-tidal values once again may not reveal how

Table 7.1 Minimal Alveolar Concentration of Inhalation Anesthetics

Anesthetic	*MAC (vol %)*
Methoxyflurane	0.16
Halothane	0.75
Isoflurane	1.40
Enflurane	1.68
Sevoflurane	1.71*
Diethyl ether	1.9
Desflurane	≈6.5*
Cyclopropane	9.2
Xenon	71
Nitrous oxide	105

Modified with permission from Eger EI II: Anesthetic uptake and action. Baltimore: Williams and Wilkins, 1976:5.

*Quoted by Eger EI II: New inhaled anesthetics. ASA Annual Refresher Course Lectures, 1989:521.

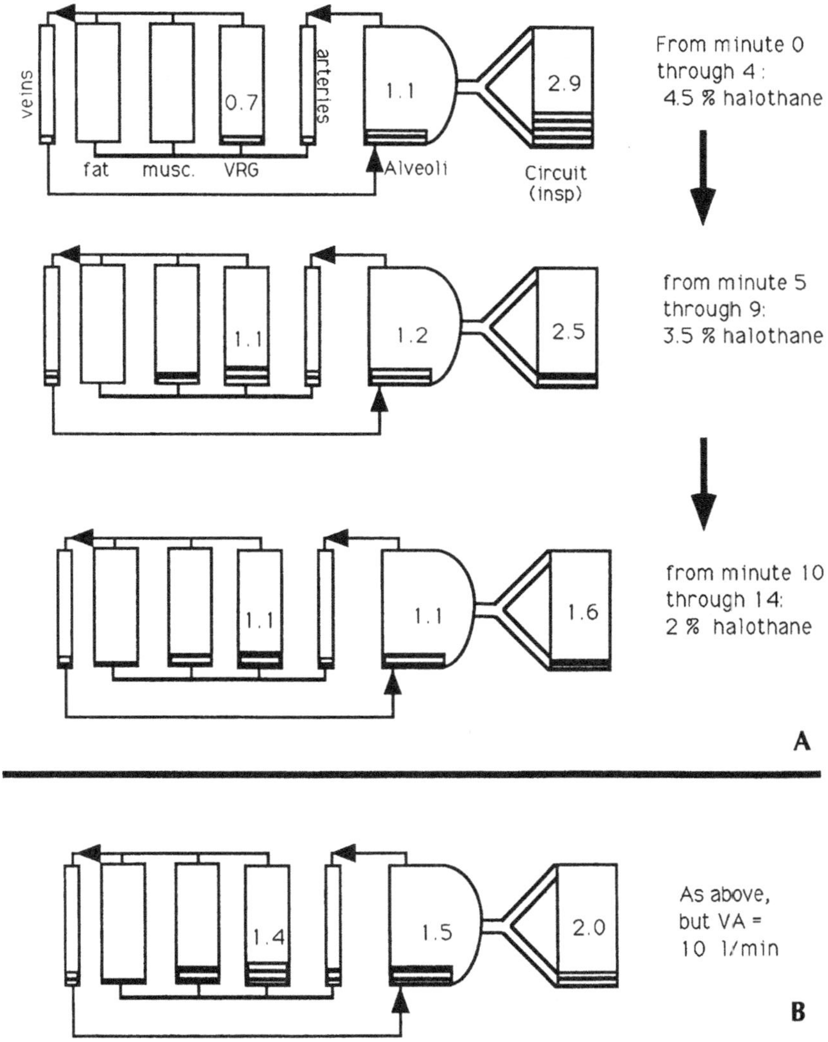

FIGURE 7.1 (A) *Anesthetic induction can start with relatively high concentrations of anesthetic agent to attain quickly the intended anesthetic partial pressure in the vessel-rich group (VRG). Shown here as an example is the administration of 4.5%, 3.5%, and 2% halothane for 5 min each. Observe that the concentrations in the alveoli and arteries reach 1.3% within 10 min, while the concentration in the VRG climbs to 1.2% only in the third 5-minute segment, when halothane had already been throttled to only 2%.* (B) *Giving a high concentration of anesthetic during induction can be dangerous. Shown is the status after 15 min of the identical induction sequence as in A, except that ventilation was increased from 4 L/min to 10 L/min. Observe that in the VRG halothane is 1.4%, which is almost 30% more than with the ventilation of 4 L/min shown in A. "Breathing a patient down" by "pumping the bag" during induction has caused cardiac arrest. These data were generated with the help of Gas Man, assuming a person weighing 70 kg and having a cardiac output of 5 L/min. Fresh gas flow was set at 5 L/min. musc. denotes muscles; insp., inspiratory.*

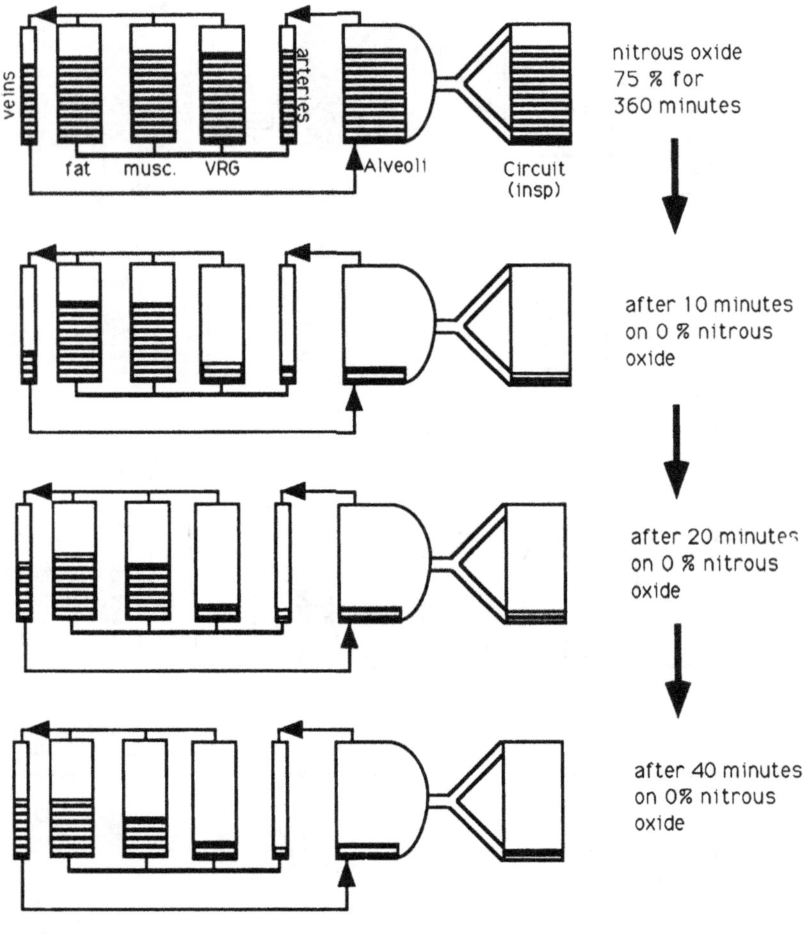

FIGURE 7.2 *After hours of anesthesia, gas tensions in the different body compartments will approach equilibrium. Observe that 75% nitrous oxide is given for 360 min and then the nitrous oxide is turned off; 10, 20, and 40 min later, the vessel-rich group (VRG) has almost no nitrous oxide, but muscle (musc.) and fat compartments still contain high concentrations. Thus, even for a relatively poorly soluble agent, the washout of anesthetic agent proceeds slowly for compartments not as well perfused as the VRG. The data were generated with the help of Gas Man, assuming a person weighing 70 kg and having a cardiac output of 5 L/min and alveolar ventilation of 4 L/min. Fresh gas flow was set at 5 L/min. insp. denotes inspiratory.*

much anesthetic has gone into solution in the organs or how long it will take to purge the body of the anesthetic agent.

For many years anesthesiologists have administered anesthetics without any information on inspired or end-tidal gas concentration. Clinical experience and the patient's responses were the only available guides to the dosing of anesthetics. With the ability to monitor anesthetic gases, the clinician has gained valuable information with which to bolster clinical impressions.

REFERENCES

1. Eger EI II: Anesthetic uptake and action. Baltimore: Williams and Wilkins, 1976:5
2. Cullen DJ: Anesthetic depth and MAC. In: Miller RD, ed. Anesthesia, vol. 1, 2nd ed. New York: Churchill Livingston, 1986:553–580
3. Silvas DL, Haynes A, Brown ACD: Potentially lethal failure of the vapor exclusion system. Anesthesiology 1989; 71:289–291

Chapter 8

The Concentration Effect, Second Gas Effect, and Diffusion Hypoxia

During induction and again during emergence from anesthesia, anesthetic gases and vapors entering and leaving the alveoli must accommodate other gases and vapors vying for the same space. The resulting shifts in concentrations of gases and vapors have consequences of clinical interest and, sometimes, importance. These consequences are the concentration effect, the second gas effect, and diffusion hypoxia. A brief discussion of these much-discussed phenomena will help the clinician appreciate the magnitude (small) and the frequency (high) of these effects.

THE CONCENTRATION EFFECT

To understand the shifts in concentrations of gases and how the inspired concentration of an inhalation anesthetic relates to the rate at which alveolar concentrations rise, imagine two alveoli, each of constant volume, as oxygen uptake is assumed to equal carbon dioxide production. Now we replace in alveolus A 8% of its volume with nitrous oxide, and in alveolus B 80% of its volume with nitrous oxide. We assume that this gas will be absorbed. The inspired tidal volume of the next breath will have to be much larger for alveolus B than A, because more gas was removed from B than A. With the next inspiration we again add a mixture containing 8% nitrous oxide in alveolus A, and 80% nitrous oxide in alveolus B. The process is repeated and we observe that the alveolar tension of nitrous oxide in alveolus B, with the higher anesthetic concentration, approaches the inspired concentration more rapidly than is true for alveolus A with the lower anesthetic concentration. This is called the concentration effect, where the patient inhales more than is exhaled. The concentration effect does not play a clinically important role with anesthetic agents that are used in low concentrations (e.g., halothane, enflurane, or isoflurane). In clinical practice, routine gas monitoring does not reveal the concentration effect (Figure 8.1).

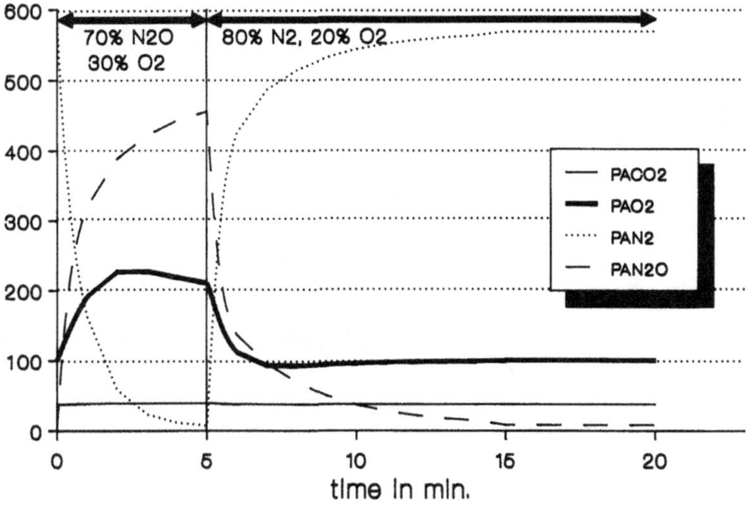

FIGURE 8.1 *The concentration effect and diffusion hypoxia. A computer plot of alveolar gas concentrations that demonstrates the wash-in and washout of nitrous oxide. Ambient pressure is assumed to be 760 mm Hg; water vapor, 47 mm Hg. From minutes 0 to 5, 70% nitrous oxide in oxygen is added to alveolar gas. The alveolar partial pressure of oxygen ($P_{A}O_2$) (heavy black line) initially overshoots its equilibration alveolar pressure because of the concentration effect. At minute 5, room air replaces nitrous oxide. The $P_{A}O_2$ now dips below its final equilibration pressure (diffusion hypoxia). $P_{A}CO_2$, $P_{A}N_2$, and $P_{A}N_2O$ denote alveolar partial pressures of carbon dioxide, nitrogen, and nitrous oxide, respectively. (Graph prepared by J.J. Heffels.)*

THE SECOND GAS EFFECT

When an anesthetic gas is sucked up and generates that extra space in the lungs into which other gases can rush, the other gases in the alveoli increase in concentration faster than would have been possible without the help of the concentration effect.[2] Thus, when isoflurane or halothane is first given, the concentration of the anesthetic increases faster during induction when a patient begins to breathe a high concentration of nitrous oxide than during anesthetic maintenance when a high concentration of nitrous oxide is in equilibrium. This is one mechanism of the second gas effect: it piggybacks the concentration effect.

There is another way of looking at the mechanisms at work. Assume that you have stabilized anesthesia with isoflurane and oxygen. Without changing the isoflurane concentration, you reduce the $F_{I}O_2$ from 1.0 to 0.3 by turning on the nitrous oxide. The nitrous oxide rushes into the blood and, thereby, reduces the volume of gas in the alveoli. This causes the isoflurane concentration in the alveoli to increase. Indeed, you may see that the inspired concentration of isoflurane momentarily falls below the end-tidal concentration of the anesthetic.[3] In other words, the concentration of the other gas (or gases) in the lung increases as another gas is taken up. The effect is not limited

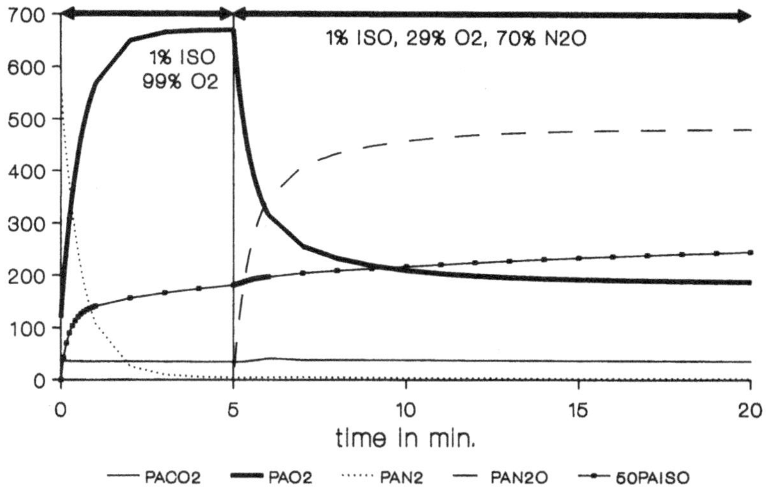

FIGURE 8.2 *The second gas effect. A computer plot of alveolar partial pressure (PA) of gases. Ambient pressure is assumed to be 760 mm Hg; water vapor, 47 mm Hg. From minutes 0 to 5, 1% isoflurane in oxygen is being added to the alveoli. At minute 5, nitrous oxide 70% replaces most of the oxygen. The alveolar partial pressure of isoflurane (PAISO) rises during the first few minutes after the introduction of nitrous oxide. In order to show the effects, the alveolar concentration of PAISO was plotted after multiplication by 50. (Graph prepared by J.J. Heffels.)*

to anesthetic agents. The same mechanism also causes oxygen and carbon dioxide to increase as nitrous oxide is introduced and absorbed (Figure 8.2).[4,5]

DIFFUSION HYPOXIA

The second gas effect describes the elimination of a gas from the lungs and the resulting changes among the remaining gases. The opposite happens at the end of anesthesia: the nitrous oxide rushes into the lung, since no additional nitrous oxide is given with the inspired gas. This nitrous oxide now filling the alveoli occupies some of the space taken up by oxygen and other anesthetics. Because in an open system the sum of all partial pressures cannot exceed ambient pressure, the appearance of a new gas must reduce the partial pressures of the other gases. If the other (diluted) gas is oxygen, and if ventilation is depressed, the patient may become hypoxemic. When the diluted gas is oxygen, the phenomenon is called diffusion hypoxia.[6] But the phenomenon is not limited to oxygen; carbon dioxide and other gases in the lung are equally affected (Figure 8.1). The patient's expired volume exceeds the inspired volume during this phase, just as the inspired volume exceeds the expired volume during induction of anesthesia with nitrous oxide.

In clinical practice, the second gas effect and diffusion hypoxia are difficult to demonstrate with routine monitoring strategies. You should be aware of these factors of gas uptake and elimination, however, and monitor oxygen saturation and the concentrations in inspired and end-tidal gases to guard against adverse events that could be attributed to these effects.

REFERENCES

1. Eger EI II: Effect of inspired anesthetic concentration on the rate of rise of alveolar concentration. Anesthesiology 1963; 24:153–157
2. Epstein RM, Rackow H, Salanitre E, Wolf GL: Influence of the concentration effect on the uptake of anesthetic mixtures: The second gas effect. Anesthesiology 1964; 25:364–371
3. Stoelting RK, Eger EI II: An additional explanation for the second gas effect. Anesthesiology 1969; 30:273–277
4. Heller ML, Watson TR Jr: The role of preliminary oxygenation prior to induction with high nitrous oxide mixtures. Anesthesiology 1962; 23:219–230
5. Kitahata LM, Taub A, Conte AJ: The effect of nitrous oxide on alveolar carbon dioxide tension: A second gas effect. Anesthesiology 1971; 35:607–611
6. Fink BR: Diffusion anoxia. Anesthesiology 1955; 16:511–519

Chapter 9

Cardiogenic Oscillations

When we speak of the inscription of the cardiac impulses on a graphic representation of gas concentration over time, the phenomenon is called cardiogenic oscillation. Every observant clinician has seen the cardiogenic play of the unidirectional valves on a circle breathing system of an anesthesia machine. During the expiratory pause, the valves are gently lifted and dropped in rhythm with the heart. These little cardiogenic breathlets occur because the right heart fills the pulmonary vascular system during systole, which forces gas out of the lungs. The vessels shrink again during diastole, and gas reenters the lungs.[1] We recorded this with the help of a volunteer who was able to keep his glottis open at the end of exhalation. He breathed through a Fleisch pneumotachograph that was set for high sensitivity. An ECG was recorded at the same time. The resulting curves (Figure 9.1) show the cardiogenic oscillations on the capnogram and the amount of air that moved with every heartbeat. In this volunteer, each heartbeat caused breathlets of about 8 ml, or about 0.1 ml/kg. At a heart rate of 60 beats/min, that amounts to a not inconsiderable minute ventilation of almost 500 ml attributable to cardiac activity. In some subjects the cardiogenic oscillations can move two to three times this volume.

Of course, even a larger volume and higher heart rate would not suffice for effective exchange of carbon dioxide and oxygen. Nevertheless, the cardiogenic ventilation plays a role in mixing gases in the lung. This was demonstrated during constant-flow ventilation, an unusual mode of ventilation during which a steady stream of gas is insufflated deep into the trachea. Cardiac arrest during constant-flow ventilation in experimental animals has reduced effective alveolar ventilation by about a third.[2] How much the heart contributes to gas exchange during spontaneous or traditional mechanical ventilation by stirring the gases in the depth of the lungs is not known. But any cardiac contribution to gas exchange gives us another reason to welcome vigorous cardiac activity.

Cardiogenic oscillations can be recorded not only at the mouth but also by sampling gas at depth in the large airways, as long as the distribution of gases in the lungs is not completely even.[3] If one pulmonary segment delivers carbon dioxide or any other gas a little earlier or later than another segment, and if the pumping activity of the heart causes the gas to shift back and forth, cardiogenic oscillations become appar-

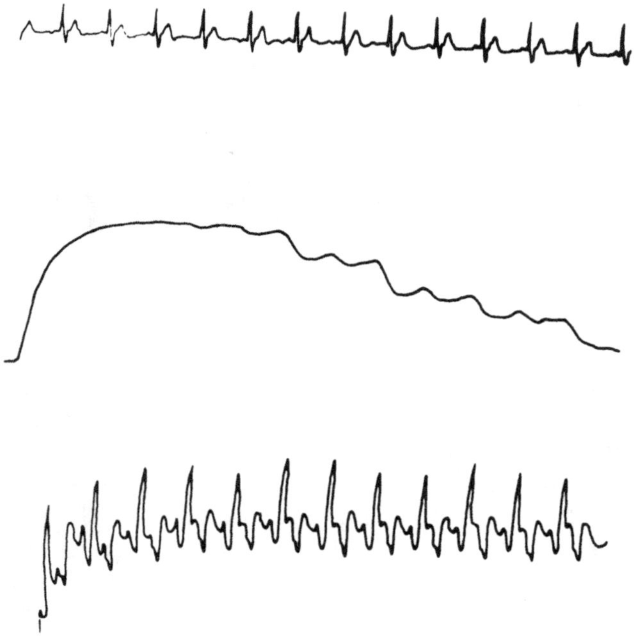

FIGURE 9.1 *Simultaneous electrocardiogram and capnogram with cardiogenic oscillations and pneumotachygram. Cardiogenic oscillations in the capnogram* (middle) *were generated from a healthy volunteer who breathed into a mouthpiece, to which a pneumotachygraph (set at high sensitivity) and sidestream capnograph sampling connector were attached. An electrocardiogram* (top tracing) *was recorded simultaneously. Oscillations appeared on the capnogram only on the downslope (phase IV). The oscillation occurred at the same rate as the heartbeat, but the two were not synchronous because of the delayed response of the sidestream capnograph, compared with the response of the pneumotachygram. In order to generate the pneumotachygram, the subject kept his glottis open after an exhalation was completed. (Reproduced with permission from Gravenstein JS, Paulus DA, Hayes TJ: Capnography in clinical practice. Stoneham, MA: Butterworths, 1989:28.)*

ent in the capnogram or the graphic representation of any other gas sampled from the carina or trachea.

Cardiogenic oscillations on recordings from gas sampled close to the mouth can be observed either because gases emerging from the trachea are still unevenly mixed, or because a sidestream analyzer aspirates some fresh gas together with the expired tidal volume from the patient while the cardiac activity superimposes small tidal volumes. Cardiogenic oscillations on an oxygram require excellent instrumentation with fast response time and brisk recording (Figure 9.2). During mechanical ventilation, cardiogenic oscillations are more readily observed with short inspirations and long expiration, for example, I:E of 1:3 rather than 1:1, and at low respiratory rates (N Gravenstein, personal communication, 1990). Cardiogenic oscillations are rarely seen in patients with severe emphysema.

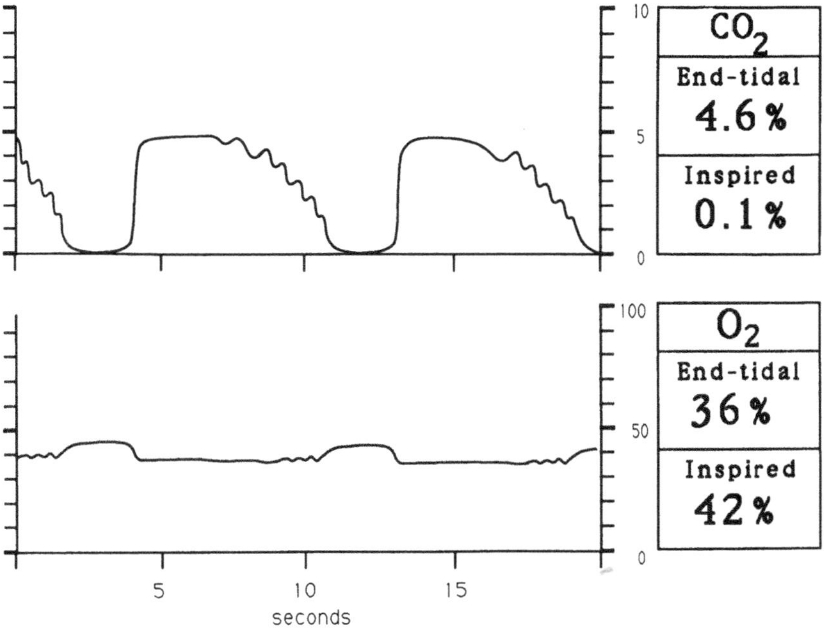

FIGURE 9.2 *Cardiogenic oscillations in a capnogram and oxygram during mechanical ventilation and endotracheal anesthesia with a narcotic and isoflurane. Recordings were made with a Brüel and Kjaer multigas analyzer.*

REFERENCES

1. Arieli R: Cardiogenic oscillations in expired gas: Origin and mechanism. Respir Physiol 1983; 52:191–204
2. Cybulsky IJ, Abel JG, Menon AS, Salerno TA, Lichtenstein SV, Slutsky AS: Contribution of cardiogenic oscillations to gas exchange in constant-flow ventilation. J Appl Physiol 1987; 63:564–570
3. Nunn JF, Hill DW: Respiratory dead space and arterial to end-tidal carbon dioxide tension difference in anesthetized man. J Appl Physiol 1960; 15:383–389

Chapter 10

Before Induction

BASELINES BEFORE INDUCTION

If we could, we would like to have a record of each patient's vital signs for the 24 preoperative hours, so that we would know that patient's normal peaks and troughs for oxygen saturation and end-tidal carbon dioxide, not to mention arrhythmias, ST depression, and arterial pressure. This would greatly help in interpreting values observed during anesthesia and after operation. How often have we collected arrhythmias during anesthesia and attributed them to the anesthetic? Yet there is good evidence that the snapshot preoperative ECG may miss major arrhythmias or ST-segment depression that the patient suffers in the course of a normal day or night.[1,2] It is reasonable to suspect that similar abnormalities occur in the realm of oxygenation and carbon dioxide homeostasis. Since we cannot afford to collect such data, we must be content with data obtained just before the induction of anesthesia. What is the oxygen saturation (SpO_2) of peripheral arterial blood according to pulse oximetry while the patient breathes room air?

Many millions of people live at altitudes of 6000 feet (approximately 2000 m) or higher and therefore breathe air with a PO_2 of around 130 mm Hg (or 17.0 kPa) or less (Table 10.1). Carbon dioxide and water vapor are added in the lungs, and PaO_2 is consequently well below 80 mm Hg, depending on barometric pressure, the state of the lungs, and to what degree hyperventilation has reduced alveolar carbon dioxide tension (P_ACO_2). A look at the oxygen dissociation curve (Figure 10.1) reminds us that under normal circumstances, the SO_2 begins to decrease steeply only as PO_2 drops below 60 mm Hg. Consequently, an SO_2 of 100% is not observed at altitudes above 6000 feet, short of introducing hypothermia or enriching the air with oxygen. Values in the mid- to low 90%s are likely.

Patients who live at high altitude merit denitrogenation with oxygen, or preoxygenation, before the induction of general anesthesia, because even mild respiratory obstruction quickly causes serious hypoxemia. Preoxygenation offers additional protection even at sea level, should the patient's airway become obstructed or should ventilation fail for other reasons. After all, the majority of disasters attributed to anesthesia have been linked to inadequate oxygenation.[3] Preoxygenation buys time.

Table 10.1 Ambient Pressure Decreases as Altitude Increases

Altitude		*Barometric Pressure*		*Oxygen Tension*		*Peripheral Arterial Oxygen Tension*
ft	*m*	*mm Hg*	*kPa*	*mm Hg*	*kPa*	*(est. mm Hg)*
Sea level		760	101	160	21.2	98
6,000	1830	609	81.2	128	17.1	93
10,000	3050	523	69.7	110	14.6	90
20,000	6100	349	56.5	73	9.8	70

Est. denotes estimated.

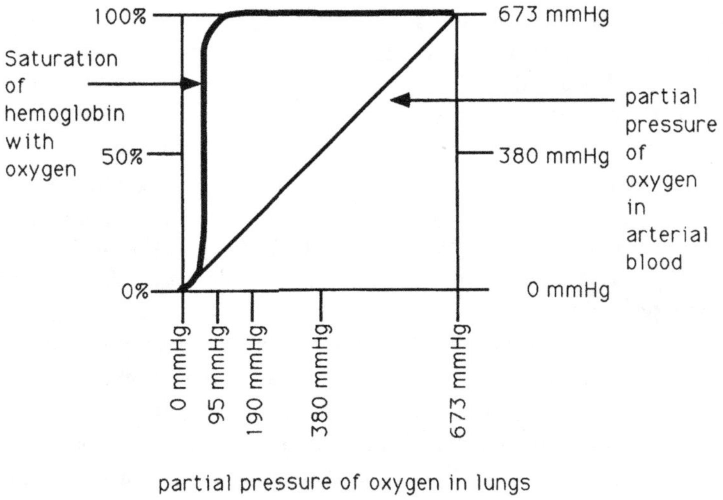

FIGURE 10.1 *The oxygen dissociation curve.*

DENITROGENATION/PREOXYGENATION

The progress of preoxygenation can be monitored in two ways. First, we can watch SpO_2. SpO_2 should rise during preoxygenation (denitrogenation) in healthy patients to about 100%, even at 20,000 feet. Looking only at SpO_2 does not enable us to determine when denitrogenation has run its course, however. We can monitor either the

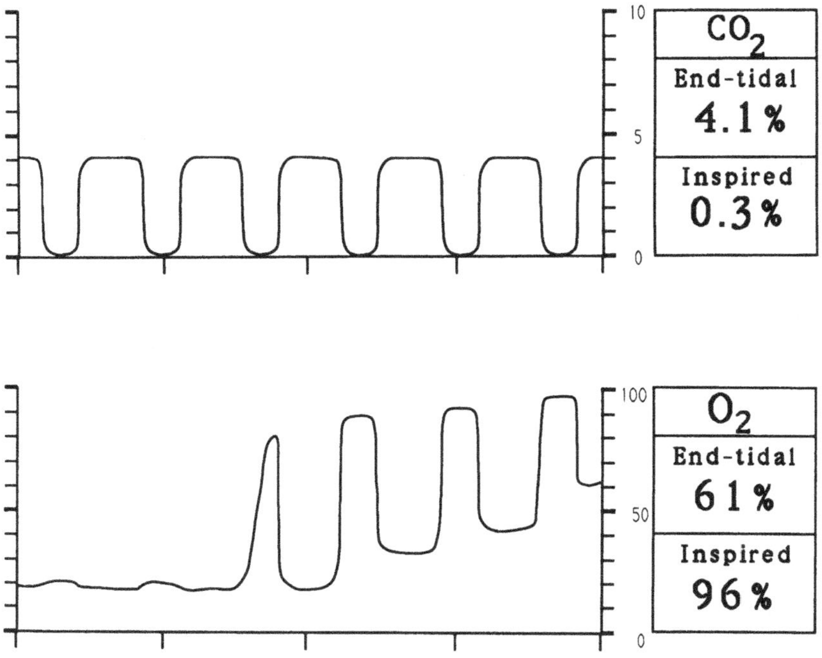

FIGURE 10.2 *Wash-in of oxygen as monitored from inspired and end-tidal gases of a patient breathing 100% oxygen from a circle breathing system. The data on the right represent the last gas concentrations determined.*

washout of nitrogen, or the wash-in of oxygen. Imagine wash-in of oxygen in a patient breathing 100% oxygen at sea level (Figure 10.2). The first few breaths cause the greatest change, and the rising curve of end-tidal oxygen grows flatter over time (Figure 10.3). The washout of nitrogen depends on the patient's pulmonary status. Many healthy patients are asked to take only three deep breaths of oxygen. In healthy volunteers, one inspiratory-capacity breath of 100% oxygen reduces end-tidal nitrogen from 80% to 75%, four breaths to 17%, and eight breaths to 6%.[4] In these subjects, end-tidal nitrogen was reduced even more with vital-capacity breaths—after four breaths to 7%, and after eight breaths to 1%.

In patients with obstructive lung disease and in the elderly, end-tidal nitrogen or oxygen may not tell the whole story; some terminal airways may be collapsed during breathing of normal tidal volumes. Deep breaths at inspiratory capacity help denitrogenation in these patients more than in the healthy, young adult. Therefore, the cautious clinician asks the patient to take many deep breaths, waits until end-tidal oxygen has plateaued, and observes with satisfaction that SpO_2 has risen to 100%.

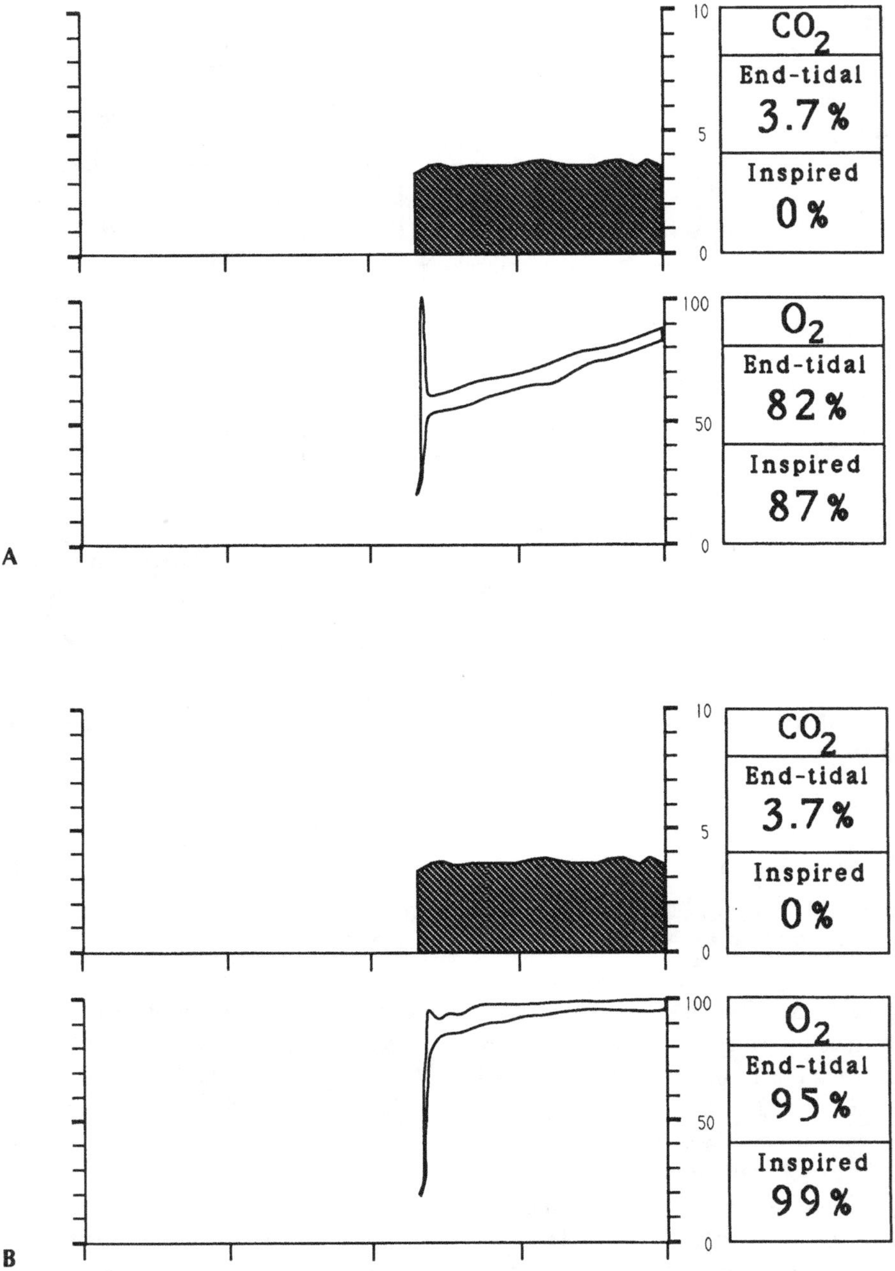

FIGURE 10.3 *Trend plot of preoxygenation.* (A) *A conscious subject is breathing into a circle breathing system with an oxygen flow of 1 L/min. Observe the slow rise of inspired and end-tidal oxygen concentrations. After 10 minutes of preoxygenation, nitrogen has not been completely eliminated from the patient's respired gas (see also Chapter 4).* (B) *The same subject during preoxygenation with a circle breathing system, but now with an oxygen flow of 6.5 L/min.*

ALARM LIMITS

Alarm thresholds on monitors should be set no later than during preoxygenation. Most devices come with default settings, alarm thresholds suggested by the manufacturer. These thresholds are not necessarily acceptable in all clinical situations.

Oxygen Analyzer Alarm Thresholds

Inspired—Low

This is the most important of all alarms. It should not be kept at the lowest value (usually 21% oxygen), but instead should be set a little below the desired FIO_2. The following case exemplifies the reason for this approach: a 50-year-old man with extensive burns undergoes operation and anesthesia with halothane and 50% nitrous oxide in oxygen. The total fresh gas flow is 5 L/min. The low alarm threshold for oxygen is set at $FIO_2 = 0.21$. Because of the burns, a pulse oximeter probe cannot be applied. Inadvertently, oxygen flow is reduced from 2500 ml/min to 250 ml/min, and the old anesthesia machine has no oxygen-proportioning device. FIO_2 slowly drops over the next several minutes; only as it falls below 0.21 does the alarm signal a low oxygen concentration. The surgeon comments that the patient's blood looks cyanotic. A short time later, the patient has a cardiac arrest. This complication would have been less likely had the anesthetist set the alarm threshold for low oxygen concentration at, say, 45%. The alarm would have been activated much earlier, and the clinician would have had ample time to pursue the necessary differential diagnostic possibilities; the patient might thus have been spared hypoxemia and cardiac arrest.

Inspired—High

When high concentrations of oxygen are hazardous (e.g., in premature newborns), the high alarm limit should be set a little above the lowest oxygen concentration at which satisfactory oxygenation can be achieved.

Carbon Dioxide

Inspired—Low

No alarm setting required.

Inspired—High

With rebreathing (see Chapter 6), inspired gas contains carbon dioxide. Because of noise and artifact, it is best to set the high alarm for inspired CO_2 above 0% (e.g., at 1%).

End-tidal—Low

Hyperventilation and other problems (see Chapters 13 and 14) can lead to low concentrations of carbon dioxide in end-tidal gas. For this, an alarm threshold may not be necessary. However, the capnograph doubles as a disconnect alarm and apnea alarm. If the capnograph fails to detect carbon dioxide, the apnea alarm should sound.

End-tidal—High

Under normal circumstances, peak P_{ETCO_2} of 45 mm Hg or 50 mm Hg are rarely exceeded. In patients in whom these values are not dangerous, high alarm thresholds at 55 mm Hg or 60 mm Hg are acceptable. In patients with hypercarbia at rest (i.e., those with chronic lung disease), higher alarm thresholds may be needed. Lower thresholds are indicated in many neurosurgical patients.

Nitrous Oxide

Alarm settings are not required because of the low potency of this agent. Excessive concentrations of nitrous oxide are dangerous because they are accompanied by low oxygen concentration. The oxygen alarms, therefore, serve in case of nitrous oxide overdose.

Anesthetic Vapors

Inspired—Low

No alarm setting necessary.

Inspired—High

When, because of malfunction or inadvertent adjustment of the vaporizer, excessive concentrations of an anesthetic vapor appear in inspired gas, an alarm should sound. Alarm thresholds can be set just above levels not exceeded in clinical practice. Because of the need to hasten induction, a relatively high concentration of anesthetic agent is often administered in the inspired gas, particularly during closed-system anesthesia. Alarm thresholds should take that into account.

End-tidal—Low

No alarm setting required.

End-tidal—High

Currently we adjust anesthetic concentrations in the fresh gas. We realize that they will not equal inspiratory concentrations (see Chapter 4) and even less so end-tidal values which are of greater concern to us (see Chapter 7). Thus, when we set the vaporizer at a certain concentration, we aim for changes in a system twice ($F_{agent\ fresh\ gas} \rightarrow FI_{agent} \rightarrow PET_{agent}$) removed. In the future we can expect systems that will adjust the concentration in fresh gas to attain the desired end-tidal values. Then alarm limits should be in force for end-tidal concentrations.

Pulse Oximetry

High

Only in patients at risk of hyperoxia (e.g., premature newborns) is it necessary to set the alarm before 100% saturation is reached. For these patients, some anesthesiologists set high SpO_2 thresholds in the low to mid-90%s.

Low

Depending on altitude and the patient's pulmonary status, pulse oximeter alarm thresholds are usually set between 85% and 90% for patients breathing room air.

Alarm technology is under close scrutiny in a number of academic centers.[5] The current crop of threshold alarms probably will be replaced eventually by more sophisticated alarm strategies. Here, artificial intelligence has a role to play. For example, rather than simply sound the alarm when a threshold is reached, it might be helpful to have the monitor check other variables before the alarm is sounded. This would reduce the incidence of false alarms, a common annoyance.

REFERENCES

1. Berger JJ, Donchin M, Morgan LS, van der Aa JJ, Gravenstein JS: Perioperative changes in blood pressure and heart rate. Anesth Analg 1984; 63:647–652
2. Eerola M, Eerola R, Kaukinen S, Kaukinen L: Risk factors in surgical patients with verified preoperative myocardial infarction. Acta Anaesth Scand 1980; 24: 219–223
3. Cheney FW: Anesthesia: Potential risks and causes of incidents. In Gravenstein JS, Holzer JF, eds. Safety and cost containment in anesthesia. Stoneham, MA: Butterworths, 1988: 11–20
4. Carmichael FJ, Cruise CJE, Crago RR, et al: Preoxygenation: A study of denitrogenation. Anesth Analg 1989; 68:406–409
5. Gravenstein JS, Newbower RS, Ream AK, Smith NT: The automated anesthesia record and alarm systems. Boston: Butterworths, 1987

Chapter 11

General Anesthesia

Regardless of the method chosen for induction of anesthesia, intubation of the trachea presents a hurdle. In completed intubation, intubation of the esophagus, or intubation of a mainstem bronchus can cause serious morbidity and even mortality. Capnography has become a trusted aid during this process. Only the lungs can deliver enough carbon dioxide to generate one capnogram after another. Therefore, a capnograph offers reliable evidence that the patient's airway, rather than the esophagus, was intubated. After esophageal intubation and ventilation of the esophagus or stomach, the capnogram is usually flat. Under exceptional circumstances, when the stomach is filled with gas containing carbon dioxide, it may maintain one or two waveforms resembling normal capnograms. However, peak end-tidal values are usually low and become successively lower with additional breaths because the stomach cannot liberate carbon dioxide as prodigiously as the lungs.

Intubation of a mainstem bronchus (Chapter 14), usually the right one, should generate lower $P_{ET}CO_2$ than tracheal intubation because the tidal volume is intended for the ventilation of both lungs. For the same reason, peak inspiratory pressure during mechanical ventilation would be elevated. However, these features would usually be observed only if the tube were first properly positioned in the trachea—with normal capnograms and normal peak airway pressure—and then slipped into a mainstem bronchus, perhaps during positioning of the patient. When the tube enters a mainstem bronchus immediately after intubation and no values for comparison are available, the resulting capnogram and peak airway pressure may seem unremarkable, and the bronchial intubation may not be recognized. In this case, pulse oximetry will signal trouble when the developing shunt reduces SaO_2 (Chapter 14).

The trachea can be intubated in a number of ways. The patient can be awake, sedated, anesthetized and breathing spontaneously, or anesthetized and paralyzed. Awake intubation carried out with a fiberoptic instrument enables the clinician to visualize the larynx and thus assure correct placement of the tube. Even here, capnography confirms that the tube has entered the trachea. For blind intubation, usually through the nose, capnography can be helpful even during placement of the tube. King and Wooten watch the capnogram with every advancement of the tube during blind nasotracheal intubation.[1]

Whether the patient is intubated or not, induction of anesthesia with inhalation anesthetics deserves a few comments. After denitrogenation, a patient's lungs are filled with oxygen, about 47 mm Hg water vapor, and about 40 mm Hg carbon dioxide. If we then prepare a new mixture that contains an anesthetic in addition to the oxygen, our attention is first drawn to the anesthesia system. We use a circle system, and we estimate its capacity to be about 7 L. To fill the system and the patient's lungs with the agent that we wish to use, we need to take the time constant into account (Chapter 4). The anesthetic will be taken up in the patient and distributed in many compartments. If our aim were to establish an equilibrium between blood and alveolar gas of, for example, 2% of an anesthetic, we would need many minutes to achieve it, if we were to begin anesthesia by using a fresh gas mixture containing 2% of the agent. Instead, most clinicians quickly increase the vaporizer setting to a much higher concentration in order to approach the desired equilibrium concentration more rapidly. Giving too much agent to the patient risks an overdose and resultant cardiac depression and even cardiac arrest, while giving too little delays induction. Being able to monitor inspired and end-tidal concentrations of anesthetics, therefore, greatly helps the clinician adjust anesthetic concentrations in the fresh gas to optimal levels.

We can induce inhalation anesthesia with one of several techniques:

1. The deep-breath technique[2]: The patient is premedicated with a narcotic to suppress the cough reflex. We equilibrate the anesthesia system with oxygen and a high concentration of one of the halogenated agents—for example, 3.5% halothane or 5% isoflurane. This represents approximately 4.5 minimum alveolar concentration for each agent. Meanwhile, from a different system the patient inhales oxygen long enough to be essentially denitrogenated. Now the patient, connected to the anesthesia system containing 5% isoflurane, is asked to exhale as much as possible and then to take a deep breath and hold it as long as possible. With this technique the patient rapidly loses consciousness after only two or three breaths, and induction of inhalation anesthesia can be continued in a routine manner.
2. After preoxygenation, the patient receives thiopental (or another rapid-acting intravenous induction agent) and a muscle relaxant. After intubation of the trachea, the administration of inhalation anesthesia is begun. In order to hasten induction, it is customary to give relatively high concentrations of the inhalation agent at this point while the patient's lungs are ventilated manually. Overdose is a danger during this rapid induction. It is therefore advantageous to monitor the inspired and end-tidal concentrations of inhalation agent.
3. After pre-oxygenation and intravenous induction, with the closed technique, the patient is connected to a circle breathing system filled with oxygen. Then, in order to bring the inspired concentration of the inhalation anesthetic to the intended level, a single dose of the liquid inhalation anesthetic is injected into the breathing circle where it vaporizes. These injections must be repeated after ever-lengthening intervals in order to maintain the level of anesthesia.[3] Even experts in this approach recommend monitoring the concentrations of oxygen and inhalation agent(s) in inspired and end-tidal gases. When using a sidestream analyzer that does not return sampled gas to the patient, the anesthetist must add enough gas to compensate for gas loss through

sampling. That may amount to between 100 and 200 ml/min. Observe that the fluctuations in inspired and end-tidal isoflurane concentrations are abrupt in a patient subjected to closed-circuit anesthesia (Figure 11.1).

4. A Mapleson system, such as the Bain or Jackson-Rees system, makes the selection of the anesthetic concentration easy, as long as the fresh gas carrying the anesthetic is inhaled by the patient without significant dilution by rebreathed gas.

Regardless of the system and the technique used, the data coming from the gas analyzer will be helpful in identifying the approach of equilibrium between inspired and end-tidal concentrations of anesthetic gas and vapor.

Emergence from anesthesia proceeds as expected; the gradients reverse themselves when we replace nitrous oxide with oxygen and as we decrease the isoflurane or similar drug (Figure 11.2 A, B, C). Now we watch end-tidal gas concentrations and estimate whether the patient will be conscious at the end of the operation or whether we need to increase the flow of fresh gas to shorten the time constants required to replace anesthetic in the circle with oxygen, lest the patient spends more time in the postanesthesia care unit while the remaining inhalation anesthetic is eliminated. The clinician must remember that end-tidal anesthetic concentrations are fed by the gases that leave the compartments of the body. Of these, the vessel-rich group (brain, heart, liver, kidney) has a high blood flow, the muscle group an intermediate blood flow, and the fat compartment a low blood flow. The longer the anesthesia has lasted, the more anesthetic agent will have equilibrated in the muscle and the fat compartments, which

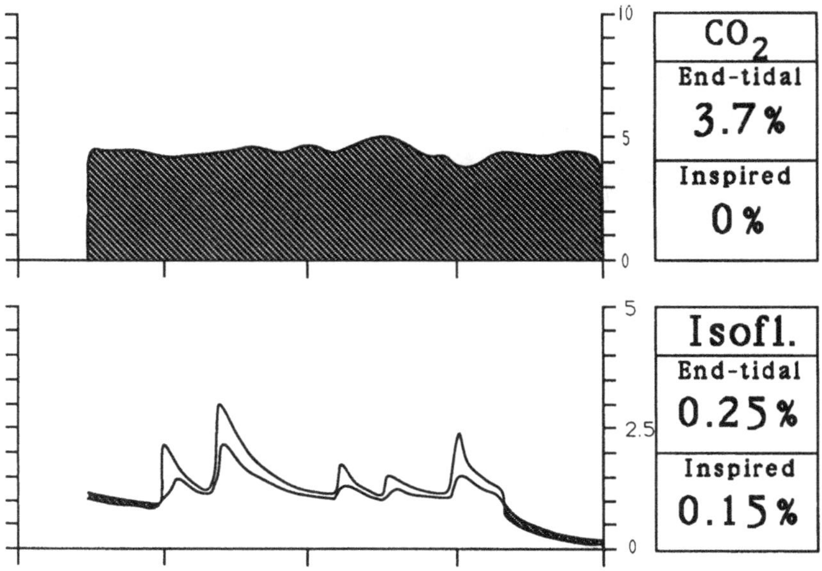

FIGURE 11.1 *With closed-circle anesthesia, inspired and end-tidal anesthetic concentrations can fluctuate abruptly. The digital data on the right represent the latest values. Isofl. denotes isoflurane.*

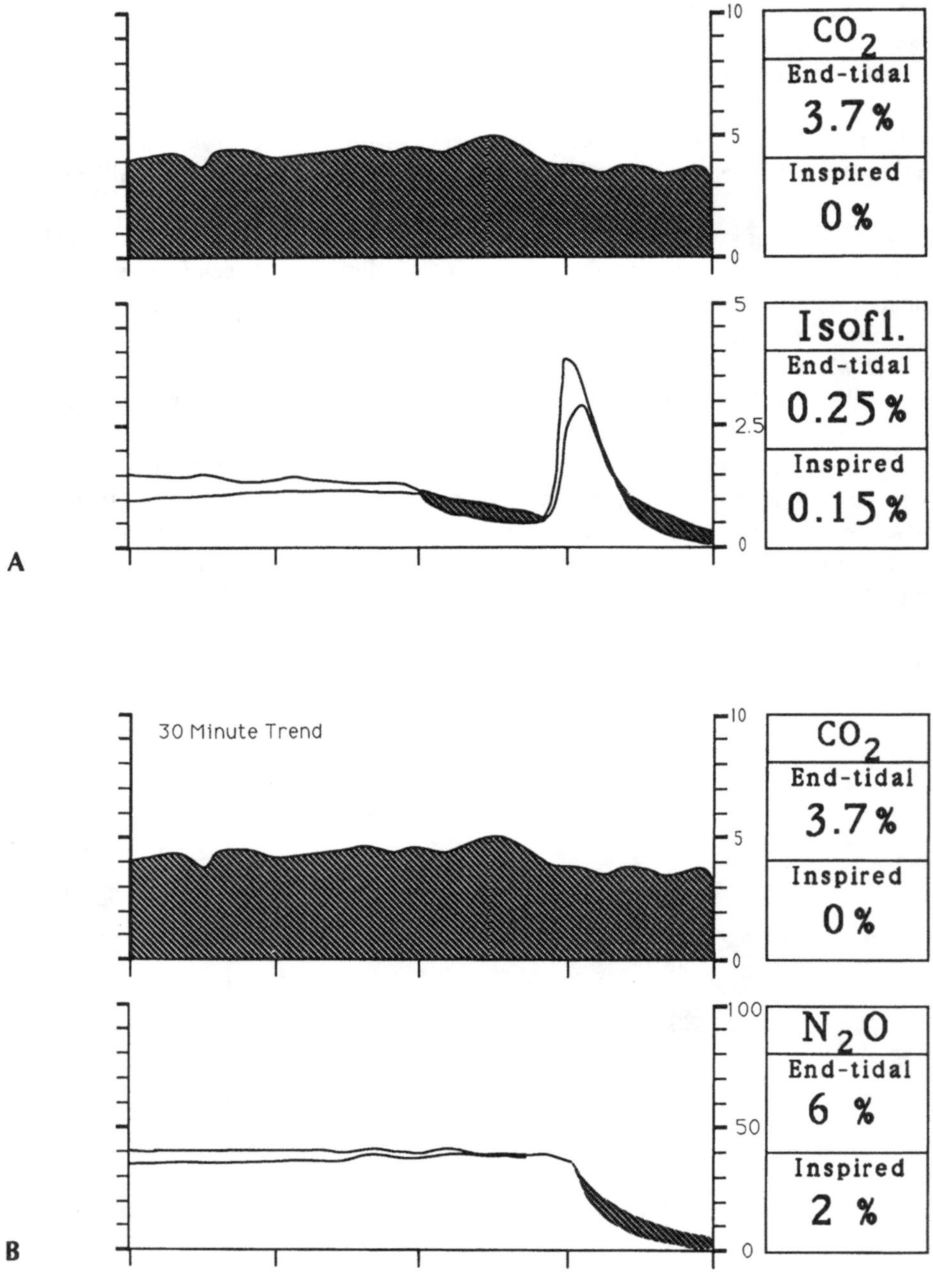

FIGURE 11.2 *The end of anesthesia. Observe that the end-tidal values of isoflurane (isofl.) and nitrous oxide exceed the respective inspired values.* (A) *At the end of anesthesia the anesthetist overestimated the speed of the surgeon, and it became necessary to deepen anesthesia briefly with isoflurane.* (B) *Once anesthesia could be discontinued, the anesthetist turned off the nitrous oxide. Observe the rapid washout of nitrous oxide.*

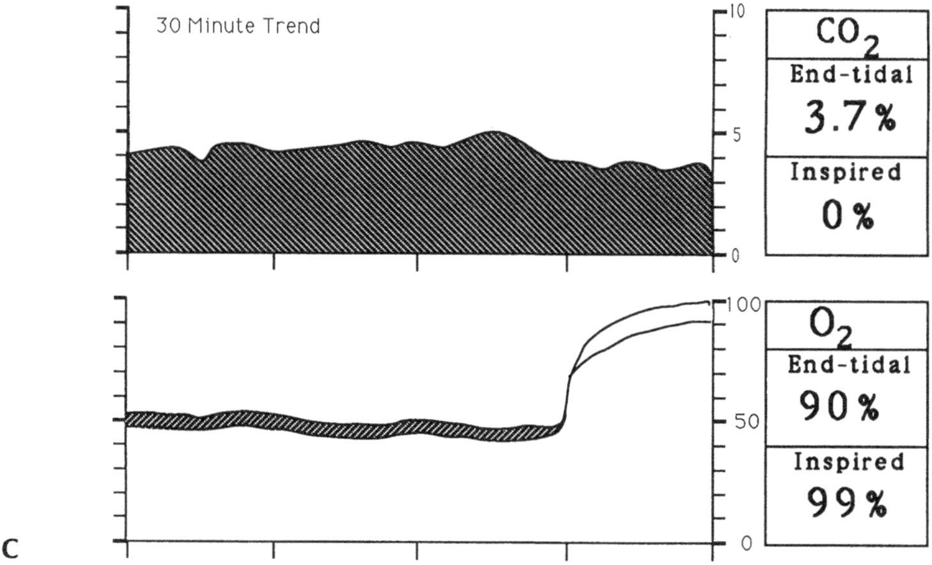

FIGURE 11.2 *(continued)*
(C) *Nitrous oxide was replaced with oxygen. Observe the trend of end-tidal carbon dioxide concentration, indicating hyperventilation during the course of anesthesia.*

have a large capacity to store the anesthetic; these compartments, therefore, will contribute anesthetic to the venous blood for some time and thus delay the decrease in alveolar gas tension. Consequently, for a given anesthetic concentration in end-tidal gas, emergence after a prolonged anesthetic takes longer than that after a brief anesthetic, all other factors being equal (see also Chapter 7).

We also keep an eye on the carbon dioxide trend plot. If we have hyperventilated the patient's lungs for hours on end, it takes time for the patient to restore the carbon dioxide level in tissue. During this time, relatively little ventilation can maintain normal $PaCo_2$ because the body absorbs some of the carbon dioxide that would have had to be exhaled if the body stores had been normal (Figure 11.3).[4,5] This relative hypoventilation has two consequences:

1. Less ventilation delays the elimination of the inhalation anesthetics. In the past—and to some degree even today—some anesthetists let the patient breathe carbon dioxide (usually 5% in oxygen) at the end of the operation in order to increase minute ventilation. In many centers this custom has fallen out of favor because a patient depressed from residual anesthetic effects has a sleepy respiratory center and is thus likely to retain carbon dioxide. To give more carbon dioxide under those circumstances appears unwise. However, if we monitor end-tidal carbon dixode levels and find them reduced in harmony with the patient's ventilation, we can administer carbon dioxide

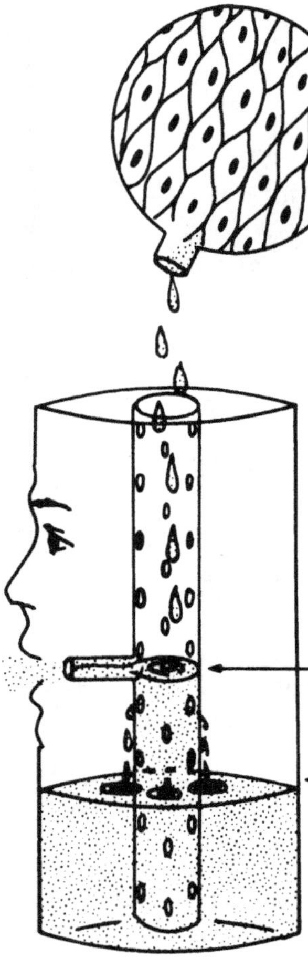

FIGURE 11.3 *Prolonged mechanical hyperventilation leads to a washout of carbon dioxide from the tissues. When the patient resumes spontaneous breathing, low minute ventilation suffices to maintain normal arterial carbon dioxide tension (PCO_2) because much of the metabolic carbon dioxide is soaked up by the tissues. The low minute ventilation may not satisfy the oxygen requirements of the body. (Reproduced with permission from Gravenstein JS, Paulus DA: Clinical Monitoring Practice. Philadelphia: Lippincott, 1987:158.)*

without concern about creating respiratory acidosis. Indeed, in order to hasten the elimination of inhalation anesthetic, we can vigorously ventilate the patient's lungs without fear of lowering $PaCO_2$ if we administer carbon dioxide in inspired gas. This should not be attempted without the use of capnography, which enables the clinician to adjust ventilation as required without fear of hyper- or hypoventilation.

2. Hypoventilation reduces the uptake of oxygen. Pulse oximetry can help ensure that the patient's SaO_2 remains normal. In addition, we can administer oxygen at the end of the operation and in the postanesthesia care unit. During hypoventilation at the

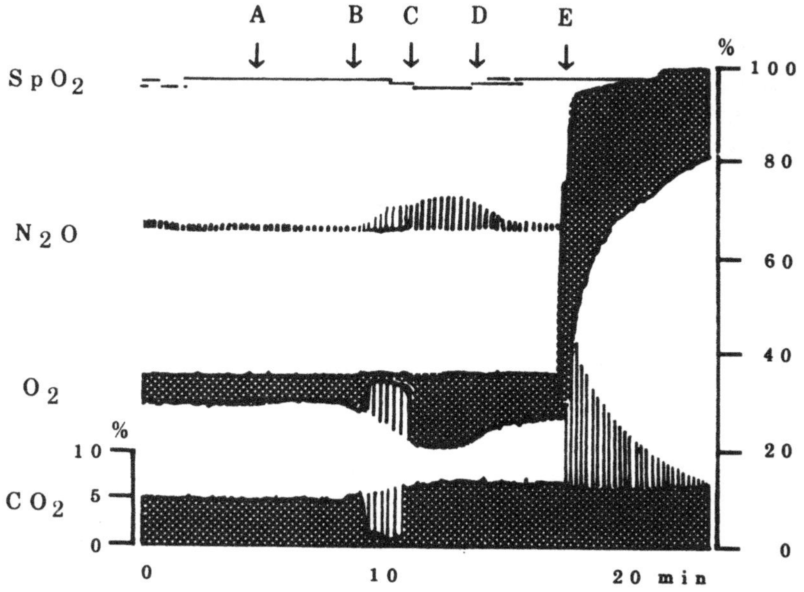

FIGURE 11.4 *Pulse oximeter readings and end-tidal gas concentrations at the end of anesthesia with a fresh gas flow of 3 L/min. Slow manual ventilation was started at B to achieve a carbon dioxide level sufficient to sustain spontaneous breathing. End-tidal oxygen changed more rapidly than did end-tidal carbon dioxide, and the difference was compensated for with the third gas, nitrous oxide. During the low end-tidal oxygen levels, pulse oximeter oxygen saturation (SpO_2) changed. At C, the patient started to breathe spontaneously. After D, alveolar ventilation and oxygen delivery were sufficient to meet the oxygen consumption, as reflected by decreasing inspiratory-expiratory oxygen and nitrous oxide differences, as well as increasing SpO_2. At E, nitrous oxide was turned off, which resulted in a rapid increase in the fraction of inspired oxygen. (Modified with permission from Linko K, Paloheimo M: Monitoring of the inspired and end-tidal oxygen, carbon dioxide, and nitrous oxide concentrations: Clinical applications during anesthesia and recovery. J Clin Monit 1989; 5:149–156.)*

end of anesthesia, the difference between inspired and end-tidal oxygen tensions increases greatly and precedes a decrease in SpO_2 (Figure 11.4).[6]

Ideally, we monitor carbon dioxide and oxyhemoglobin percentage and keep them normal and monitor the levels of anesthetics in respired gas and see that they are close to zero at the end of the operation.

REFERENCES

1. King H-K, Wooten DJ: Blind nasal intubation by monitoring end-tidal CO_2. Anesth Analg 1989; 69:412–413
2. Loper K, Reitan J, Bennet H, Benthuysen J, Snook L Jr: Comparison of halothane and isoflurane for rapid anesthetic induction. Anesth Analg 1987; 66:766–768

3. Lowe HJ, Ernst EA: The quantitative practice of anesthesia: Use of closed circuit. Baltimore: Williams and Wilkins, 1981
4. Salvatore AJ, Sullivan SF, Papper EM: Postoperative hypoventilation and hypoxemia in man after hyperventilation. N Engl J Med 1968; 280:467–470
5. Postoperative hypoxemia—another cause. N Engl J Med 1969; 280:503 (editorial)
6. Linko K, Paloheimo M: Monitoring of the inspired and end-tidal oxygen, carbon dioxide, and nitrous oxide concentrations: Clinical applications during anesthesia and recovery. J Clin Monit 1989; 5:149–156

Chapter 12

Pulse Oximetry and Monitoring of Gases in Patients under Regional or Local Anesthesia with or without Sedation

Many patients undergo local or topical anesthesia and sedation without being monitored during operative or diagnostic procedures. This can be quite safe as long as the patient is not seriously ill, the operator or examiner does not interfere with the patient's ventilation, and the local anesthetic causes no toxic or allergic reaction. As long as the patient answers questions, one may assume that cerebral perfusion and oxygenation are adequate. Indeed, the give-and-take of conversation makes for an inexpensive, sensitive, and continuous assessment of cerebral function.

Two changes in the patient's condition should alert the clinician to the possibility of problems: the patient becomes restless or the patient falls asleep. One often follows the other, particularly when the restless patient has been given depressant medication. Restlessness is dangerous because it may signal cerebral hypoxia, onset of a toxic reaction to the local anesthetic, or an overdose of vasopressors administered together with the local or topical anesthetic. Many serious complications have arisen when restlessness was not interpreted as a sign of trouble; instead, it was assumed that the patient was simply apprehensive, uncomfortable, or in pain. Then sedative, hypnotic, anxiolytic, or narcotic drugs were administered intravenously. The patient fell asleep, and the underlying problem was exacerbated by the depressant effects of the medication. All too often, respiratory arrest followed.

A restless patient under local, topical, or regional anesthesia demands careful attention. Before depressant drugs are given, the patient should be examined, and problems other than anxiety and pain should be ruled out. If depressant drugs are given intravenously, I recommend that a formal monitoring protocol be instituted. This can consist of conversation with the patient. If the patient does not respond well to conversation, additional monitoring should be begun. Depending on the patient's general health, this may include regular determination of BP, an ECG, pulse oximetry, and even capnography. All of these monitors can be set to collect data automatically and to sound an alarm when preset limits are exceeded.

CAPNOGRAPHY

Because many patients receive oxygen by face mask or nasal prongs during regional or local anesthesia, ventilation can be monitored with the help of capnography. Several methods of sampling end-tidal gas from a patient who is not intubated have been described. A sampling catheter can be taped to the chin of a patient whose face is covered by drapes (Figure 12.1)—for example, during eye operations under retrobulbar block. An alternative is to insert a catheter into one of the prongs of the nasal oxygen assembly and aspirate gas from there (Figure 12.2), as described by Bowe et al.[1] One can also insert the sampling catheter about 1 cm into a nostril or cover the tip of a soft tube with a piece of soft plastic foam. This end is inserted in one nostril, the other connected to the capnographic sampling catheter.[2] It is helpful to cut a hole into the side of the tip of the catheter that rests in the nostril; this prevents obstruction of the tip with nasal mucosa. Any of the methods will give information at least on the frequency of ventilation—valuable information should the patient be at risk of hypoventilation.

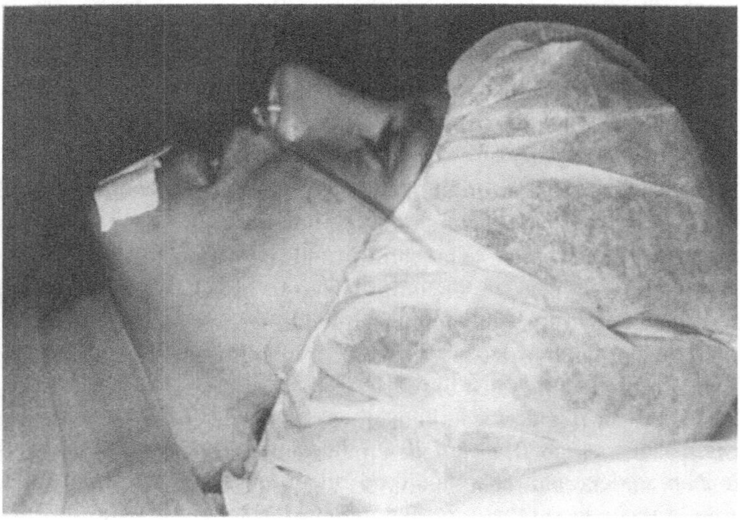

FIGURE 12.1 *The sampling capillary for respiratory gas monitoring can be taped to the chin when a patient's face will be covered by drapes (e.g., during an ophthalmic operation.)*

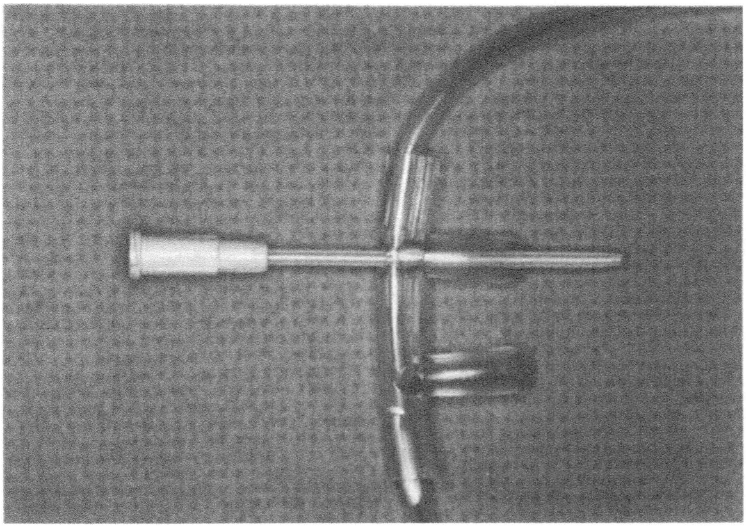

FIGURE 12.2 *The sampling catheter for respiratory gas monitoring can be attached to an intravenous catheter that has been inserted into one prong of nasal oxygen prongs.*

When the patient's face is covered by drapes, capnography also enables the clinician to gauge the adequacy of gas exchange under the drapes. The dead space that is formed by the drapes will result in an accumulation of carbon dioxide and a lowering of oxygen concentration in the inspired gas. It is easy to route fresh gas under the drapes and monitor the concentrations of inspired carbon dioxide and oxygen.

OXIMETRY

In a patient undergoing excision of a pilonidal cyst under spinal anesthesia (Figure 12.3), the collecting capillary was inserted into one prong of the nasal cannula, and 3 L/min of oxygen was blown into the nasal prong.

PULSE OXIMETRY

What has been said for capnography also applies to oximetry. As soon as centrally active medication to allay the patient's fears has been administered, and as soon as the patient becomes sleepy or dozes off, additional monitoring is indicated. As our ultimate concern lies with hypoxia, pulse oximetry serves well for these patients. Not only can

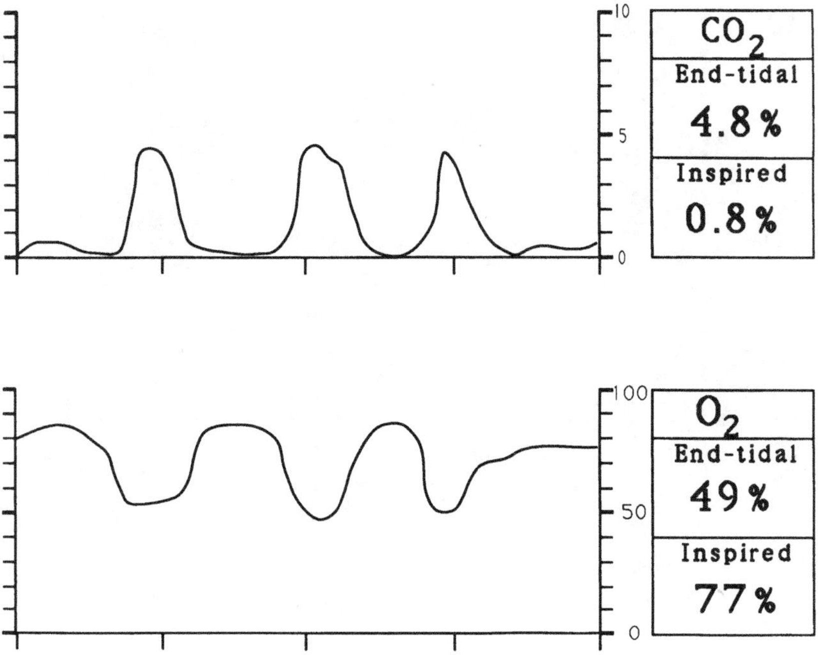

FIGURE 12.3 *To monitor respiratory gases in a patient under regional anesthesia, gas was aspirated from one nasal prong.*

we discover the onset of hypoxemia, but we have information on oxygenation as well as pulse rate, and we have one measure of peripheral perfusion. Should the pulse oximeter fail to detect a pulsatile signal in the periphery, the patient should be examined for circulatory difficulties.

In patients breathing room air, decreasing saturation, as monitored with the pulse oximeter, must cause concern. The physician needs to consider hypoventilation if $PaCO_2$ is increasing or a shunt is developing—for example, as with beginning atelectasis from bronchial obstruction. The effect of carbon dioxide retention on alveolar, and consequently arterial, oxygen concentration can be illustrated with the help of the alveolar gas equation:

$$P_{A}O_2 = (760 - 47) \times 0.21 - \frac{40}{0.8},$$

or in words: the partial pressure of alveolar oxygen tension ($P_{A}O_2$) equals the barometric pressure (here 760 mm Hg) minus the pressure of water vapor in the alveoli (here 47 mm Hg assuming a temperature of 37.1 °C) multiplied by the fraction of inspired oxygen (here room air with an $F_{I}O_2$ of about 0.21). From this value we subtract the PCO_2 in equilibrium with arterial blood (here assumed to be 40 mm Hg) corrected for the respiratory quotient (here assumed to equal 0.8). Although this idealized equation does not do justice to the inevitable shunts that serve to make P_AO_2 less than PaO_2, the equation is helpful in visualizing the impact of changes in P_ACO_2; the point deserves emphasis, because the PaO_2 calculated with this ideal equation is likely to be higher—by an unpredictable amount—than P_AO_2.

In the above example the P_AO_2 would equal almost 100 mm Hg. SpO_2 would be close to 100%. Now assume that because of respiratory depression the $PaCO_2$ were to double under one of two conditions: breathing room air or breathing 50% oxygen:

With room air:

$$(760 - 47) \times 0.21 - \frac{80}{0.8} = P_AO_2 \text{ of } 49.7 \text{ mm Hg}$$

With 50% oxygen:

$$(760 - 47) \times 0.5 - \frac{80}{0.8} = P_AO_2 \text{ of } 256.5 \text{ mm Hg}$$

When room air is breathed, the patient's SpO_2 would decrease to about 80%; when 50% oxygen is breathed, SpO_2 would still be 100%. Thus, when giving oxygen to the patient, do not assume that all is well just because the patient's blood is well oxygenated. Some clinicians do not enrich the air with oxygen in a conscious patient (under regional or local anesthesia) *whose hemoglobin is well saturated* so that the first decrease in SpO_2 can reveal a respiratory depression, which calls into action whatever measures are needed to diagnose the problem and correct it. To help with the diagnosis in such a case one might ask the patient to breathe through a mouthpiece connected to the gas sampling catheter of a gas analyzer that has a rapid response time and can record both $P_{ET}O_2$ and $P_{ET}CO_2$. Respiratory depression is reflected by a $P_{ET}O_2$ lower than normal for the patient's F_IO_2 and a correspondingly high $P_{ET}CO_2$.

Forced to rank monitors for patients under regional or local anesthesia, I would list the pulse oximeter ahead of all others because it gives almost heartbeat-to-heartbeat information on oxygen saturation and heart rate. Of course, in patients at risk from cardiovascular complications, oximetry should be joined by the measurement of BP and the ECG. Cardiovascular complications can arise if the patient has heart disease or hypertension or if the clinician interferes with the cardiovascular system. For example, blocking sympathetic nerves during spinal or epidural anesthesia renders the patient more vulnerable to hypotension, and blocking the accessory muscles of ventilation increases the risk of hypoventilation. Spinal and epidural anesthesia are quite safe, but disasters do happen.[3] Cardiac arrest during spinal anesthesia can occur fairly suddenly. One well-documented cardiac arrest during spinal anesthesia was recorded with the help of an automated anesthesia record-keeping system (Figure 12.4). The clinicians were pleased that they could document that hypoxia—a preventable cause of arrest—had not been a factor leading to this patient's trouble. The patient was well monitored, the physicians responded quickly and successfully, and the patient survived a potentially lethal complication.

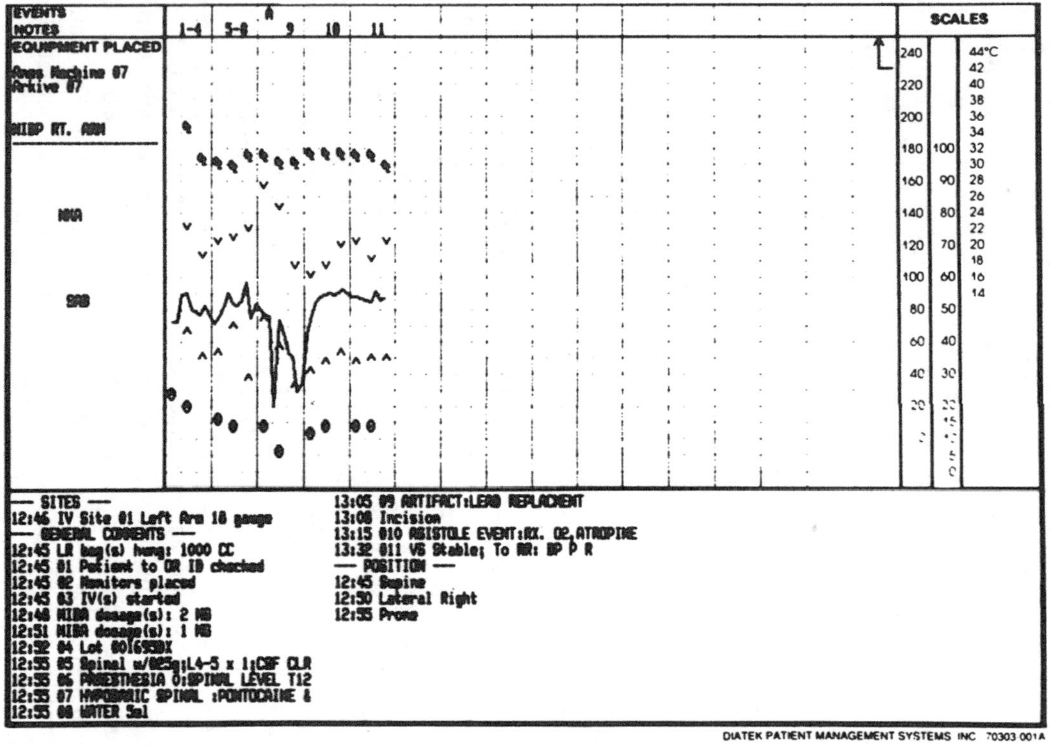

FIGURE 12.4 *Cardiac arrest during regional anesthesia was well documented by means of an automated anesthesia record-keeping system. Observe that the normal pulse-oximetry data suggests that a mechanism other than hypoxia led to the arrest. The patient was resuscitated and recovered well after the operation. (Courtesy of David W. Edsall, M.D., Chairman, Department of Anesthesiology, Burbank Hospital, Fitchburg, MA.)*

REFERENCES

1. Bowe EA, Boysen PG, Broome JA, Klein EF Jr: Accurate determination of end-tidal carbon dioxide during administration of oxygen by nasal cannulae. J Clin Monit 1989; 105–110
2. Bonsu AK, Tamilarasan A, Bromage PR: A nasal catheter for monitoring tidal carbon dioxide in spontaneously breathing patients. Anesthesiology 1989; 71:318
3. Caplan RA, Ward RJ, Posner K, et al: Unexpected cardiac arrest during spinal anesthesia: A closed claims analysis of predisposing factors. Anesthesiology 1988; 68:5–11

Chapter 13

Metabolic Changes

The availability in the operating room and postoperative stations of means to measure oxygen and carbon dioxide in inspired and end-tidal gas has opened up new diagnostic opportunities. Long before a drift in temperature alerts the clinician to a change in the basal metabolism of a patient requiring mechanical ventilation, a trend in P_{ETCO_2} and in the ratio between inspired and end-tidal oxygen concentrations can point to altered metabolism. The indications are indirect and must be interpreted with caution for two reasons. For one, as long as we see only the concentration but not the amount of oxygen absorbed or carbon dioxide eliminated per minute, we cannot measure metabolic variables. For another, in the operating room we are often dealing with unsteady states. Even if one had data on the amount of gas consumed or eliminated per minute, the fact that one might be looking at transient disturbances would make interpretation difficult. Nevertheless, we need to be aware of what processes might be at work when we observe that the ratio of inspired to end-tidal oxygen has changed or that the P_{ETCO_2} has gone up or down. Before discussing some of the more common conditions under which basal metabolism is affected, a few words about respiratory quotient and metabolic rate.

DEFINITION OF RESPIRATORY QUOTIENT

Oxygen taken up by the lungs finds its way into the cells, where it fuels a complex metabolic factory that generates energy and carbon dioxide. Carbon dioxide, in turn, leaves the cells and travels in blood back to the lungs, from which the gas is exhaled. Measurement of the amount of oxygen taken up and the amount of carbon dioxide produced provides a glimpse at the nature of metabolism.

In general, about 20% more oxygen is consumed than carbon dioxide produced. The ratio of carbon dioxide production to oxygen consumption is called the respiratory quotient (RQ). It varies with the substrate burned in the cellular factory. Compared with the metabolism of glucose with a respiratory quotient of 1.0, the metabolism of lipids lowers the RQ to about 0.7. The RQ for the metabolism of protein lies between that of carbohydrates and lipids.

DEFINITION OF METABOLIC RATE

When we discussed the ratio of carbon dioxide production to oxygen consumption, we looked at the quotient without worrying about the amount of oxygen consumed or the amount of carbon dioxide produced. However, these amounts give an indication of the rate of metabolism in general. Metabolic rate is usually expressed in terms of calories or joules (1 calorie [written with a lowercase *c*] = 4.18 joules = the amount of heat required to warm 1 g of water from 15 °C to 16 °C) or kilocalories (1 kilocalorie = 1 Calorie [written with a capital *C*] = 1000 calories). The basal metabolic rate is measured in Calories per hour. The average adult at rest consumes about 1 Calorie per hour per kg body weight, a figure easy to remember. For an adult weighing 70 kg, the daily consumption would be around 1680 Calories (70 × 24) at rest. No wonder that many diets call for a cutback of caloric intake to about 1800 Calories per day, without curtailment of activities!

With each liter of oxygen, about 4.8 Calories are consumed. Assuming an RQ of 0.85, this can be restated for carbon dioxide: each liter of exhaled carbon dioxide reflects the consumption of about 5.6 Calories. The metabolism of 1 g mole of glucose generates about 686 Calories. That is, 1 g of glucose generates about 3.8 Calories; 1 L of 5% dextrose in water therefore generates about 190 Calories.

GLUCOSE INFUSION AND RESPIRATORY QUOTIENT

As long as oxygenation and acid-base balance remain normal, ventilation is driven by the carbon dioxide tension in blood. If carbon dioxide production falls, ventilation can be throttled. That is of some interest in patients with respiratory insufficiency who need to exert great effort to maintain normal PCO_2 in blood, or in whom mechanical ventilation cannot keep up with carbon dioxide elimination. Giving these patients glucose and thus raising the RQ causes greater demand for ventilation than does maintaining an RQ close to 0.7.

During anesthesia, glucose is often administered intravenously, together with balanced salt solutions. In patients receiving glucose during anesthesia, the RQ in the recovery room was above 0.9, and the average carbon dioxide production was 175 ml/min. Compare that with patients given only balanced salt solution during anesthesia: RQ in the recovery room was below 0.8, and average carbon dioxide production was 150 ml/min.[1]

ANESTHETIC EFFECTS ON METABOLIC RATE

Offhand, one would assume that metabolism could never be lower—given the same body temperature—than during general anesthesia, and particularly during mechanical ventilation of a paralyzed patient. Interestingly enough, in animal studies, the lowest basal metabolic rates have been observed during normal unmedicated sleep, when oxygen consumption fell to 2.5 ml/kg/min, whereas it rose during general anesthesia to

3.5 ml/kg/min with mechanical ventilation and to 4.5 ml/kg/min with spontaneous ventilation.[2]

EFFECT OF BODY TEMPERATURE

Patients are often exposed to a cold operating room during anesthesia. Opening a body cavity particularly accelerates the loss of heat by evaporation and convection. The intravenous infusion of cold solutions exacerbates cooling. Mild hypothermia, therefore, is common in modern anesthesia. In particular, small children, who have large body surface areas for their weights, can cool quickly. They may not have the strength to shiver postoperatively, which would elevate temperature again, or to breathe normally. Hypothermia, therefore, must be prevented. With hypothermia in the anesthetized patient comes a reduction in oxygen consumption and carbon dioxide production. A rule of thumb suggests that every decrease (or increase) by 1 °C will decrease (or increase) oxygen consumption—and, hence, carbon dioxide production—by about 7%. This would call for an equal reduction in ventilation in order to avoid inducing hyperventilation in the hypothermic patient. This rule of thumb works only for a physiologic range of temperature between about 30 °C and 40 °C.

The question of what constitutes a normal carbon dioxide level during hypothermia or hyperthermia has not been answered satisfactorily. A sensible suggestion is to check arterial blood gases. Before analysis under anaerobic precautions, the blood should be warmed (or cooled) to a temperature of 37 °C. If blood gas values at this normalized temperature are normal, ventilation was properly adjusted.

MITOCHONDRIAL DEFECTS

That thyroid disease can alter basal metabolism is well known. Rarely do patients with untreated thyroid dysfunction undergo elective operation. In an emergency, however, we may encounter such patients. Hyperthyroidism elevates oxygen consumption and carbon dioxide production, and hypothyroidism does the opposite. I assume that thyroid dysfunction will be evident in the patient's history and physical examination well before we can deduce metabolic abnormalities from monitoring oxygen and carbon dioxide in respired gas. If we harbor suspicions, we might examine the ventilator settings required to maintain what appear to be normal carbon dioxide and oxygen levels in the expired gas. In a supine, anesthetized, paralyzed patient with normal lungs, normal body temperature, and normal lean body mass, a mechanically delivered tidal volume of about 10 ml/kg body weight with 10 breaths/min should bring $P_{ET}CO_2$ into the neighborhood of 32 mm Hg to 39 mm Hg. If $P_{ET}CO_2$ deviates grossly from this norm, the clinician will be justified in searching for a reason, one of which might be mitochondrial defects. Much more likely, and diagnostically more readily interpreted, are changes in $P_{ET}CO_2$ that evolve during anesthesia. External cooling or heating or endogenous hypermetabolism must then be suspected.

MALIGNANT HYPERPYREXIA

In patients genetically predisposed to malignant hyperpyrexia, a triggering substance such as succinylcholine or halothane can cause the basal metabolism to increase to a frightening degree. Eventually the heart rate accelerates, the body temperature rises, and metabolic acidosis supervenes. However, before acidosis can develop and before body temperature can rise, the cellular mechanism must be pushed to generate the extra energy, which entails burning more oxygen and producing more carbon dioxide. Monitoring $P_{ET}CO_2$ has therefore proven to be a sensitive and early indicator of malignant hyperpyrexia. In a 4-year-old boy under halothane anesthesia after endotracheal intubation with the help of succinylcholine,[3] it took 2 h before the patient began to hyperventilate and before $P_{ET}CO_2$ increased from 30 mm Hg to 90 mm Hg. By that time, his temperature had increased only from 35.2 °C to 37 °C. Malignant hyperpyrexia was diagnosed, and the patient was treated successfully with dantrolene and supportive measures.

REFERENCES

1. Hagerdal M, Caldwell CB, Gross JB: Intraoperative fluid management influences carbon dioxide production and respiratory quotient. Anesthesiology 1983; 59:48–50
2. Mikat M, Peters J, Zindler M, et al: Whole body oxygen consumption in awake, sleeping and anesthetized dogs. Anesthesiology 1983; 58:18–25
3. Dunn CM, Maltry DE, Eggers GWN Jr: Value of mass spectrometry in early diagnosis of malignant hyperthermia. Anesthesiology 1985; 68:333

Chapter 14

Ventilation-Perfusion Inequalities

Gas monitoring and pulse oximetry do not relieve the clinician of the responsibility to check arterial and perhaps mixed venous blood gases when ventilation-perfusion inequalities are suspected. For isolated estimates of mixed venous PCO_2 ($P\bar{v}CO_2$), one can have the patient rebreathe a concentration of carbon dioxide that is a little higher (by about 20 mm Hg) than that assumed to exist in the mixed venous blood (D. Thomson, personal communication, 1989). The technique calls for only a bag, a mask (or a fitting for an endotracheal tube), and a capnometer. If the patient's $P\bar{v}CO_2$ is assumed to be around 6 volume percent, the 3-L bag is filled with a 9% mixture of carbon dioxide in oxygen. The patient is then made to rebreathe the mixture in the bag for three deep breaths in order to bring the gas in the lung close to equilibrium with the gas in the bag. The equilibrated gas in the bag is then analyzed in a capnometer. The result should be close to that for mixed venous blood. The technique presupposes a steady state and conditions that enable the clinician to estimate the $P\bar{v}CO_2$ before making the measurement.

If the differences between venous and arterial, between arterial and alveolar, and between alveolar and end-tidal gas tensions were always predictable, life would be simple (Figure 14.1). But they are not. This chapter discusses broadly why the differences between end-tidal and alveolar gas tensions and between end-tidal and arterial gas tensions change. Increased differences carry important clinical information, as they give evidence of ventilation-perfusion (V/Q) inequalities (Figure 14.2). We discover these only when we have obtained blood for analysis of gases and compare these results with the tensions of respired gases.

WHEN TO SAMPLE ARTERIAL BLOOD FOR GAS ANALYSIS

The clinician will need to obtain arterial blood and have it analyzed for gas tensions if the tensions of expired gases or the oxygen saturation appear inappropriate for the patient's ventilation, inspired oxygen concentration, or both.

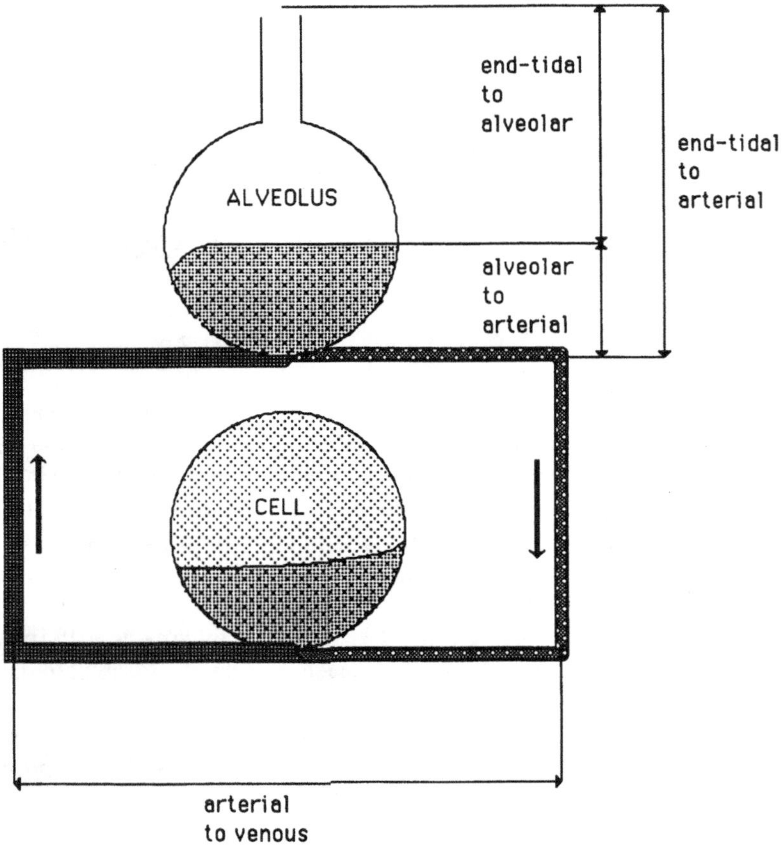

FIGURE 14.1 *Differences between end-tidal, alveolar, arterial, and mixed venous gas tensions. The alveolar tension cannot be measured, and the mixed venous rarely is. End-tidal tensions may not reflect alveolar, arterial, or venous values.*

Inappropriate Ventilation

Under ideal circumstances, the $P_{ET}CO_2$ and $P_{ET}O_2$ mirror $PaCO_2$ and PaO_2. Small discrepancies in PCO_2 values ($PaCO_2$ minus $P_{ET}CO_2$) of 4 mm Hg to 6 mm Hg are explained by anatomic shunts (e.g., the Thebesian veins) and some physiologic mismatch of V/Q of alveoli.[1] However, under some circumstances the differences can grow much larger. Such increased differences must be suspected when the minute ventilation appears to be inappropriate for a given patient. Normally, we expect a tidal volume of about 10 ml/kg body weight and a respiratory rate of 10 breaths/min to bring end-tidal values into a physiologic range.

Malfunction of the equipment must be ruled out. For example, a cracked gas-sampling capillary may cause room air to be aspirated along with a patient's gas. Abnormally low $P_{ET}CO_2$ will be the result. At other times the ventilator setting appears

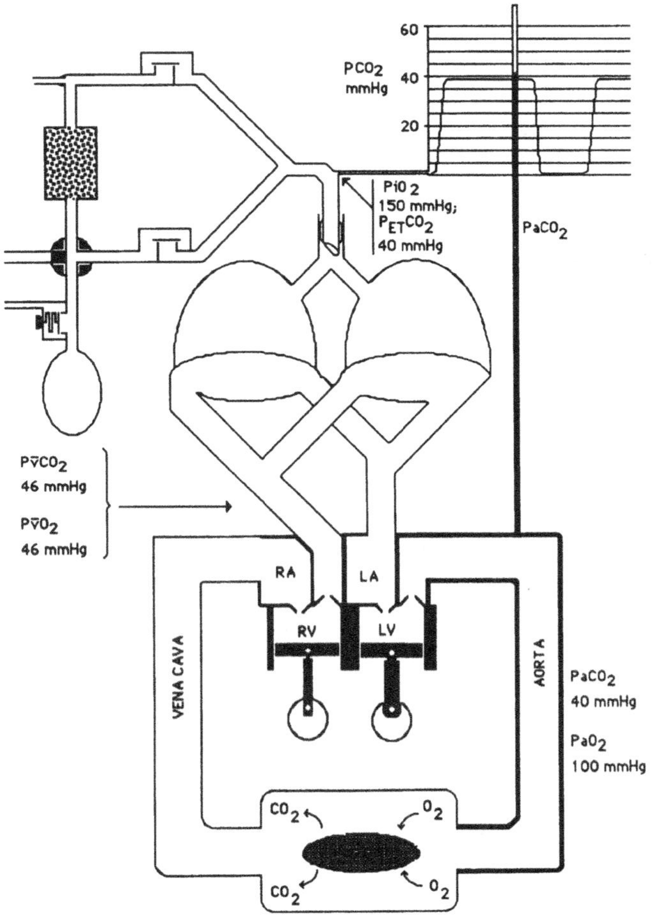

FIGURE 14.2 *Schematic presentation of the respiratory and cardiovascular systems. An endotracheal tube is in place and attached to an anesthesia circle-breathing system. The aorta is catheterized to measure arterial carbon dioxide tension ($PaCO_2$), the value of which is superimposed on a capnogram obtained from a sampling site close to the endotracheal tube. ET denotes end-tidal, I, inspiratory; $\bar{v}$, mixed venous; RA and LA, right and left atrium; RV and LV, right and left ventricle.*

to be appropriate and end-tidal gas tensions seem normal, yet arterial gas tensions are abnormal.

Abnormal Saturation

In clinical practice the pulse oximeter often gives the first hint that something is amiss with alveolar ventilation, perfusion, peripheral circulation, or all of these. Such indications are more likely when the inspired gas mixture contains less than 100% oxygen.

Desaturation is common during general anesthesia, when perfusion and ventilation of different lung fields become mismatched because of mechanical ventilation, the lateral body position of the patient, or anesthetic depression of pulmonary vascular reflexes that normally contribute to the proper matching of perfusion to ventilation. Concerns about desaturation usually overshadow worries about the $PaCO_2 = PACO_2$ difference. The clinician may be aware of these possibilities or may be taken by surprise. In case of desaturation, one first rules out mechanisms that would point to difficulties with the anesthesia machine, ventilator, gas delivery, and minute ventilation. By far the most common problem during general anesthesia, however, stems from a mismatch of ventilation and perfusion, often abetted by hypotension and a low cardiac output.

INADEQUATE VENTILATION

Despite proper settings of the ventilator, ventilation of the patient's lungs may be inadequate.

Esophageal Intubation

Intubation of the esophagus instead of the trachea continues to rank as one of the most common errors leading to disaster in anesthesia. Many methods have been advocated to assure proper positioning of the endotracheal tube in the trachea. One of the best is capnography. A normal capnogram followed by others that look no different from the first affirms that the tube is in the correct place. If the tube winds up in the esophagus (or the mediastinum), an extreme pulmonary V/Q mismatch exists (i.e., there is no pulmonary ventilation).

Endobronchial Intubation

A typical V/Q mismatch develops with inadvertent intubation of one mainstem bronchus and the subsequent ventilation of only one lung (Figure 14.3). To prevent unintentional intubation of a mainstem bronchus, we auscultate over both lung fields while inflating the lungs by compressing the breathing bag. When a cuffed endotracheal tube has been placed, one can also palpate the cuff through the trachea between larynx and jugular notch by placing two or three fingers along the trachea and inflating and deflating the cuff. With a properly positioned tube, one can easily feel, through the trachea, the swelling of the cuff. As long as it is detected below the larynx and above the jugular notch, one can rest assured that the tip of the tube has not slipped past the carina. After testing for the position of the cuff, do not leave the cuff inflated more than necessary to prevent a gas leak during peak inspiratory pressure.

When the cuff cannot be palpated and auscultation of the lungs renders ambiguous information, diagnosis becomes more difficult. Respired gases may not give a clear indication either, as end-tidal values for the ventilated lung can be normal even though

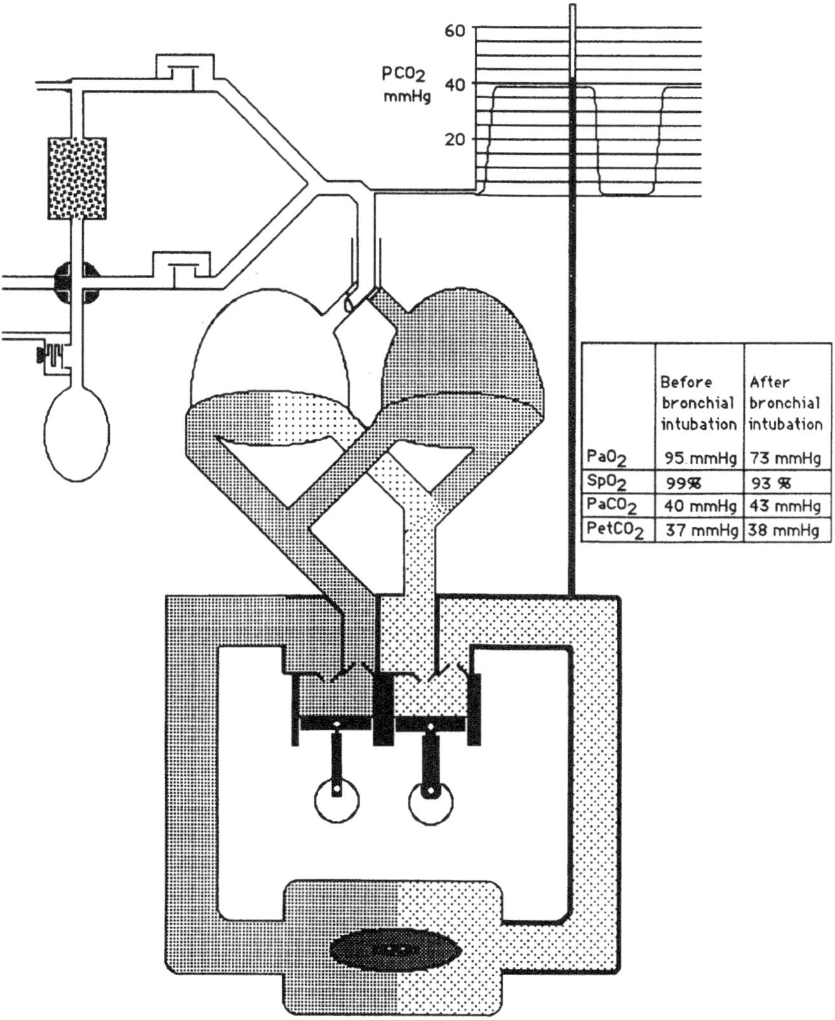

	Before bronchial intubation	After bronchial intubation
PaO_2	95 mmHg	73 mmHg
SpO_2	99%	93 %
$PaCO_2$	40 mmHg	43 mmHg
$PetCO_2$	37 mmHg	38 mmHg

FIGURE 14.3 *With bronchial intubation, only one lung is ventilated. Possible gas tensions in arterial and peripheral arterial blood (PaO_2, $PaCO_2$) and end-tidal (P_{ETCO_2}) gas are shown before and after bronchial intubation. The pulse oximeter oxygen saturation (SpO_2) may decrease unless the patient is breathing a high concentration of oxygen. Similar findings may follow bronchial obstruction with mucus or aspiration of a foreign body. (See Figure 14.2 for explanation of the schematic representation.)*

it should be relatively hyperventilated. But eventually the pulse oximeter often reveals the problem (Figure 14.3). The large shunt will affect PaO_2 more than $PaCO_2$ because the normal difference between $P\bar{v}O_2$ and PaO_2 is large, while the normal difference between $P\bar{v}CO_2$ and $PaCO_2$ is small. Mixing equal parts of venous blood with arterial blood will therefore affect oxygen more than it will carbon dioxide. Monitoring

PaO_2 would generate the first data that would lead the clinician to consider endobronchial intubation.[2] However, the pulse oximeter alarm will also sound if FIO_2 is not high enough to prevent desaturation after a large shunt.

Bronchial or Airway Constriction

If expiration proceeds slowly and, before it has run its course, is interrupted by the next inspiration, end-tidal values will not reflect alveolar values. This observation is common in patients with asthma or other conditions with bronchiolar, bronchial, tracheal, or endotracheal tube narrowing. Phase III and often even phase II of the capnogram appear sloped (Figure 14.4).

INADEQUATE PERFUSION

Low Cardiac Output

If low cardiac output fails to deliver enough oxygen to the tissue and venous blood returns to the lungs with a high carbon dioxide concentration, removing this carbon dioxide load from the reduced blood flow through the lungs is readily accomplished with normal ventilation. End-tidal and arterial values for carbon dioxide and oxygen tensions may look normal, or nearly so. Under these conditions it is advantageous to obtain mixed venous blood to assess tissue levels of carbon dioxide, pH, and PO_2. In a study of patients with circulatory failure, arterial blood gas values were often quite normal because of vigorous mechanical ventilation. The inadequacy of circulation and the futility of the treatment, however, became apparent on inspection of central venous blood samples (Table 14.1).[3] Neither end-tidal nor arterial values of carbon dioxide and oxygen tensions indicated the inadequacy of tissue perfusion under circumstances of cardiac failure or arrest. Unfortunately, the continuous monitoring of mixed venous blood is not a noninvasive routine. Typically, even with a sudden cardiac arrest, washout of carbon dioxide does not cease from one breath to the next. Instead, $PETCO_2$ decreases with every breath as carbon dioxide is slowly washed out from blood that is stagnating in the lungs and from the lung tissue itself. Cardiac arrest has a more rapid effect on the difference between inspired and end-expired oxygen tension; the two values approach equilibrium faster than is true for carbon dioxide, because blood and tissue store little oxygen.

Obstructed Pulmonary Blood Flow

If segments of the pulmonary artery are occluded—for example, with an embolus (air, clot, or tumor) or by a surgical maneuver—some alveoli are ventilated but not perfused (Figure 14.5). These alveoli constitute an alveolar dead space. The gas ventilating the

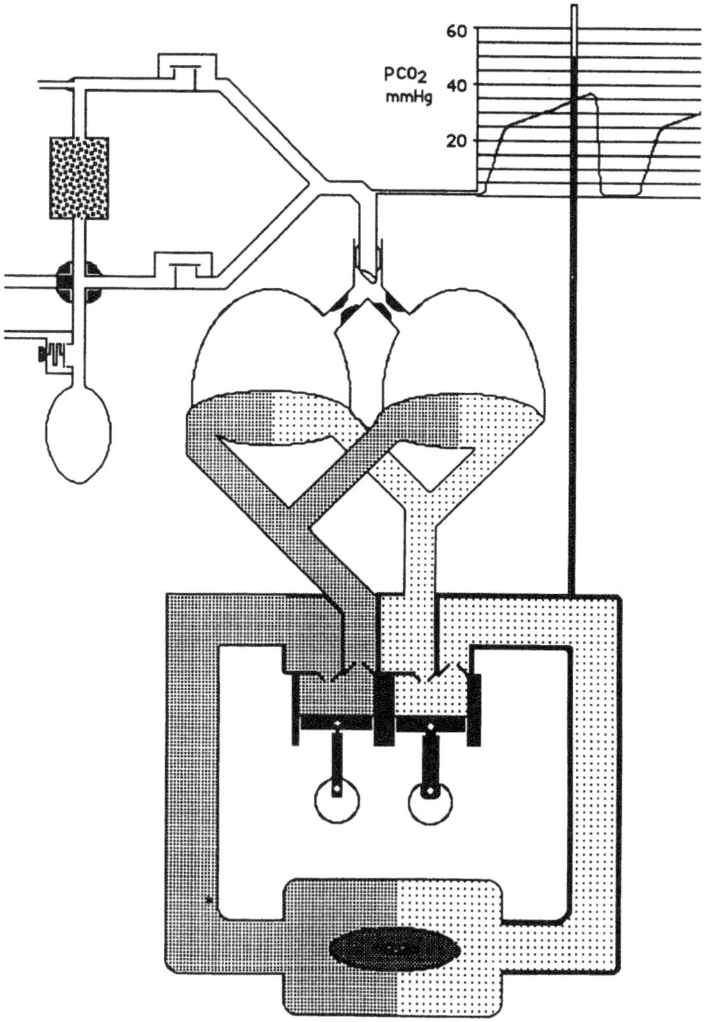

FIGURE 14.4 *Airway narrowing—for example, with asthma or chronic obstructive lung disease—causes typical sloping in phases II and III of the capnogram. Expiration is prolonged, and inspiration may be initiated before expiration has run its course. This results in a large difference between end-tidal and arterial values for carbon dioxide (PCO_2) and oxygen tensions. (See Figure 14.2 for explanation of schematic representation.)*

unperfused segments is expired without having delivered oxygen and without having taken up carbon dioxide. End-tidal carbon dioxide concentration will therefore be lower, and the end-tidal oxygen concentration higher than normal. The typical observation of decreasing end-tidal carbon dioxide concentration during otherwise steady-state

Table 14.1 Arterial Blood Gas Values in Patients in Circulatory Shock

	Blood Gas Values During Various Circulatory States			
	*Normal**	*Mild Reduction of Cardiac Output†*	*Severe Circulatory Failure*	*Cardiac Arrest with Mechanical Ventilation*
pH				
Arterial	7.38	7.39	7.31	7.36
Central venous	7.35	7.33	7.21	7.01
PCO_2 (mm Hg)				
Arterial	37	36	43	27
Central venous	43	43	68	76
PO_2 (mm Hg)				
Arterial	300	302	80	116
Central venous	64	59	30	17

*Cardiac indexes > 2.5 L/min/m^2.

†Cardiac indexes of 1 to 2.5 L/min/m^2.

Modified with permission from Adrogué HJ, Rashad MN, Gorin AG, et al: Assessing acid-base status in circulatory failure. Difference between arterial and central venous blood. N Engl J Med 1989; 320: 1312–1316.

anesthesia raises the suspicion of an increased alveolar dead space. The difference between $P_{ET}CO_2$ and $PaCO_2$ will be increased.

With air embolism pulmonary blood flow is often only partially obstructed.[4,5] Air bubbles lodge in the pulmonary vascular bed and nitrogen from them goes into solution and then diffuses into the alveoli. Detecting nitrogen in the end-tidal gas, therefore, will be pathognomonic for air embolism. Three caveats:

With sidestream analyzers a small leak in the sampling capillary will cause nitrogen to appear in the respired gas. The values should be similar in inspired and end-tidal gas, provided the patient had been denitrogenated.

A leak in the breathing circuit will admit air and thus nitrogen, but only if the intraluminal pressure becomes negative during part of the respiratory cycle, as with ventilators with hanging bellows, for example.

Not all proven pulmonary air embolisms lead to detectable nitrogen in the end-tidal gas. Sometimes nitrogen emerges only fleetingly and is missed; often its concentration is too low to be detected by the commercially available clinical gas analyzers.[6]

Anatomic Shunts

Some blood is shunted past the alveoli. When such shunts become large—for example, during surgical manipulation of the lungs—the physiologic differences between end-tidal and arterial gas tensions can increase dramatically (Figure 14.6).

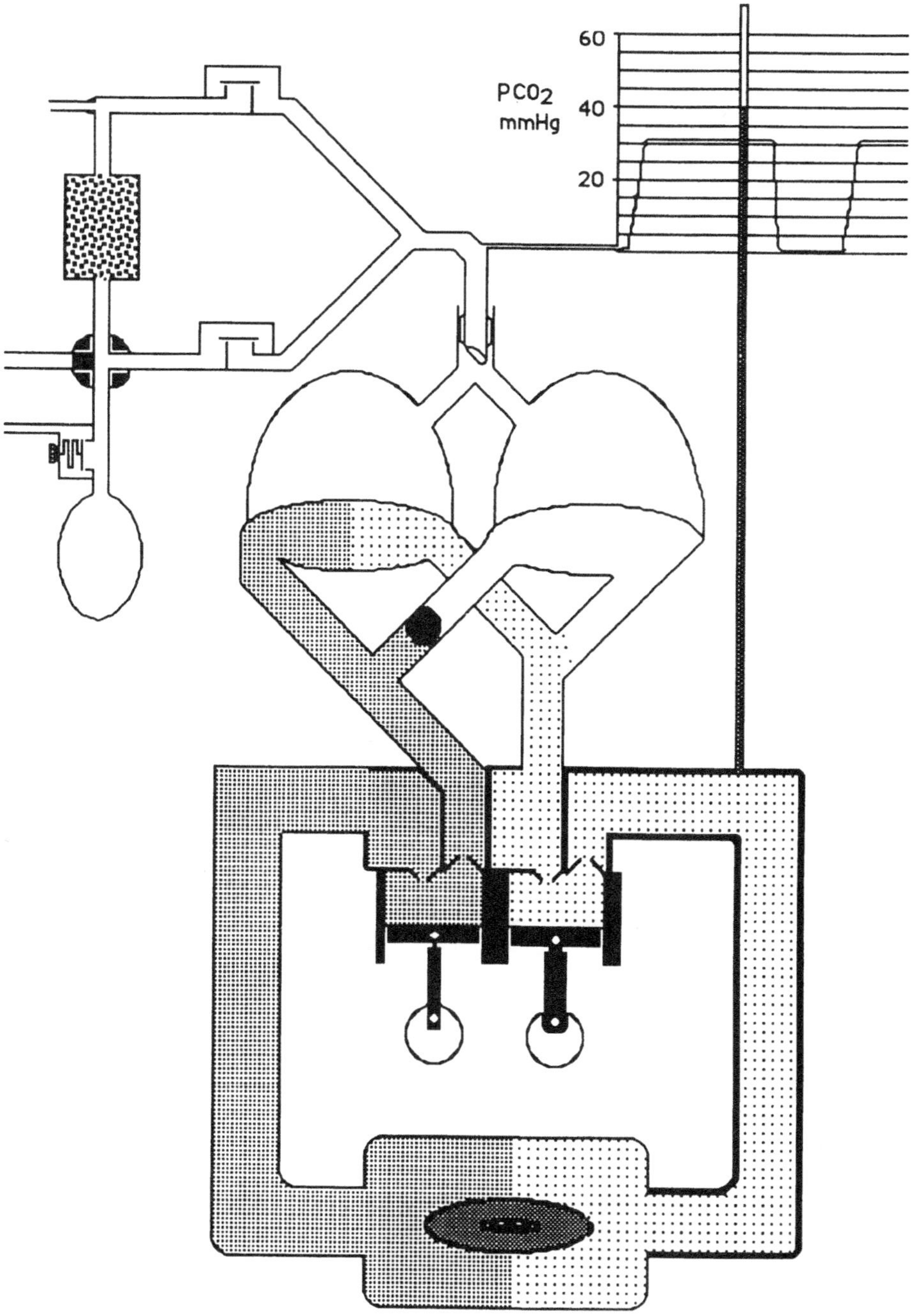

FIGURE 14.5 *Obstruction of a pulmonary artery with an embolus, tumor, air, or surgical maneuver results in futile ventilation of the unperfused lung. This alveolar dead space causes a large difference between arterial and end-tidal values for carbon dioxide tension (PCO_2). (See Figure 14.2 for explanation of the schematic representation.)*

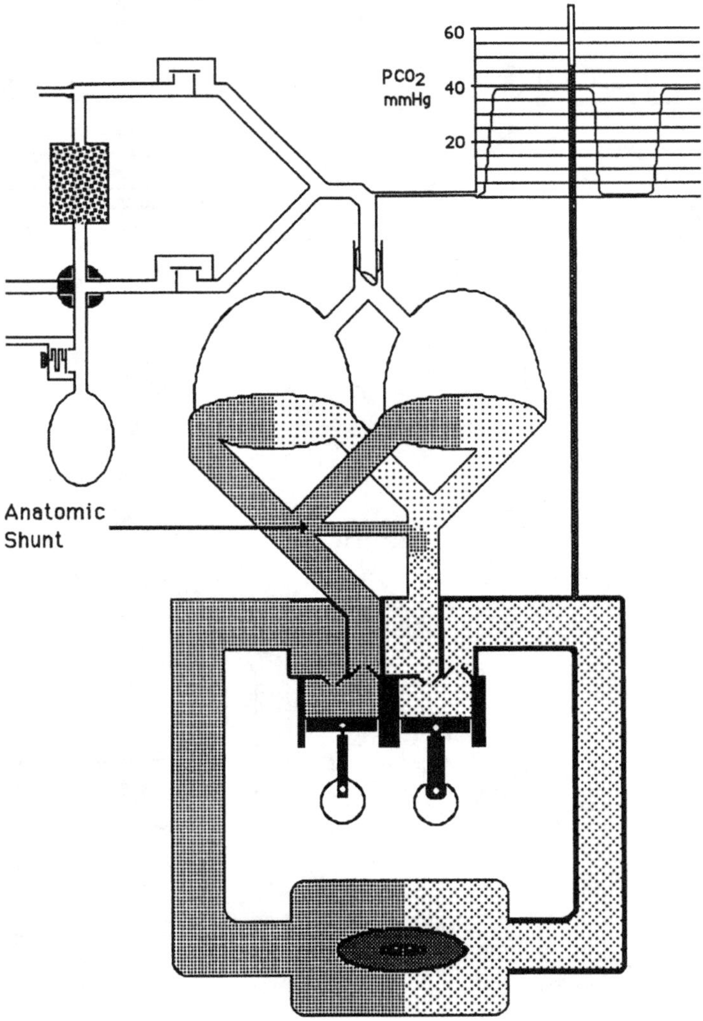

FIGURE 14.6 *An anatomic shunt shuttles blood past the alveolus and thus lowers arterial oxygen (PaO_2) and increases arterial carbon dioxide ($PaCO_2$) tensions. The shunt affects PaO_2 more than $PaCO_2$. (See Figure 14.2 for explanation of the schematic presentation.)*

REVERSED GRADIENT

Occasionally $P_{ET}CO_2$ exceeds $PaCO_2$ (Figure 14.7). We know that there must be large fluctuations of carbon dioxide concentration in the alveoli as fresh gas comes into equilibrium with alveolar capillary blood. We assume that these fluctuations are reflected in the arterial blood—probably significantly damped, but measurable. By obtaining an arterial blood sample during the nadir of $PaCO_2$, the $P_{ET}Co_2$ can be

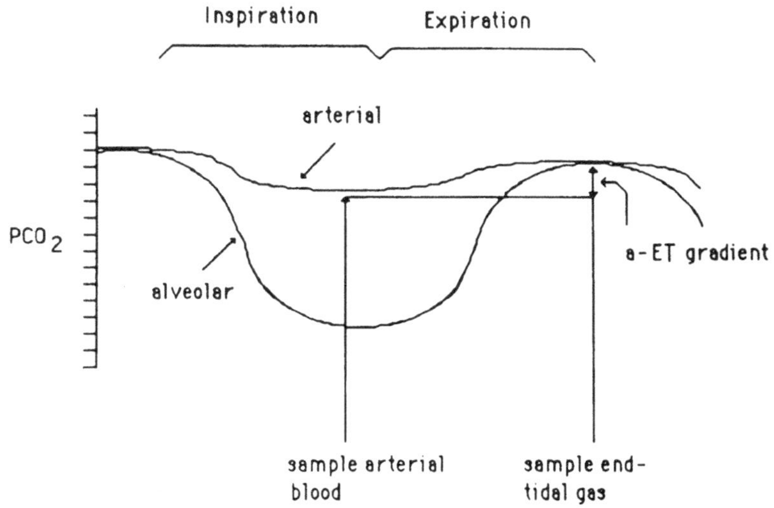

FIGURE 14.7 *Diagrammatic presentation of the fluctuations of alveolar and arterial carbon dioxide tension (PCO_2) during a respiratory cycle. When these fluctuations are large, it is likely that some samples will show the end-tidal (ET) to exceed arterial (a) PCO_2, as would have happened if samples had been obtained as indicated in the diagram.*

higher than the $PaCO_2$. It is understandable, then, that such a reversed gradient will be more likely when alveolar fluctuation of $PaCO_2$ is wide, as would be true in a patient with large tidal volume for a given functional residual capacity (e.g., a pregnant patient).[7,8]

SUMMARY

A check of $PaCO_2$ and PaO_2 will show an enlarged difference between arterial and end-tidal partial pressures when V and Q are mismatched. The diagrams of V/Q mismatch do not do justice to the usual clinical circumstances. V/Q abnormalities rarely are attributable to a single cause. The surgeon's work in the chest often complicates matters even further. The best the clinician can do is monitor gases, watch the pulse oximeter, and draw arterial blood for gas analyses by which to compare arterial to end-tidal values and thus obtain a clue about the status of V/Q matching.

This discussion of V/Q inequalities has dealt exclusively with oxygen and carbon dioxide. However, if an unexpected increase in the difference between end-tidal and arterial gas tensions exists for the physiologic gases, the same will apply for the anesthetic agents; their gradients would run parallel, or nearly so, to those for oxygen during induction of anesthesia and those for carbon dioxide during emergence from anesthesia.

REFERENCES

1. West JB (ed): Ventilation blood flow and gas exchange, 3rd ed. Oxford, England: Blackwell Scientific Publications, 1970
2. Barker SJ, Temper KK, Hyatt J, Heitzmann H: Comparison of three oxygen monitors in detecting endobronchial intubation. J Clin Monit 1988; 4:240–243
3. Adrogue HJ, Rashad MN, Gorin AB, Yacoub J, Madia NE: Assessing acid-base status in circulatory failure: Difference between arterial and central venous blood. N Engl J Med 1989; 320:1312–1316
4. Verstappen FTJ, Bernards JA, Kreuzer F: Effects of pulmonary gas embolism on circulation and respiration in the dog. III. Excretion of venous gas bubbles by the lung. Pflügers Arch 1977; 370:67–70
5. English JB, Westenskow D, Hodges MR, Stanly TH: Comparison of venous air embolism monitoring methods in supine dogs. Anesthesiology 1978; 48:425–429
6. Matjasko J, Petrozza P, Mackenzie CF: Sensitivity of end-tidal nitrogen in venous air embolism detection in dogs. Anesthesiology 1985; 63:418–423
7. Shankar KB, Moseley H, Kumar Y, et al: Arterial to end-tidal carbon dioxide tension difference during Caesarean section anaesthesia. Anaesthesia 1986; 41:698–702
8. Fletcher R, Johnson B: Deadspace and the single breath test for carbon dioxide during anaesthesia and artificial ventilation. Br J Anaesth 1984; 56:109–119

Chapter 15

Methods of Gas Analysis

In anesthesia we are dealing with the physiologic gases (oxygen, carbon dioxide, nitrogen, and water vapor) and the anesthetic gases and vapors. In the last decades a number of methods of analyzing these anesthetic agents almost continuously in respired gas have reached such maturity that today one can buy quite reliable equipment for this purpose—equipment that also analyzes physiologic gases. New methods for gas analysis continue to appear. The following discussion examines the cardinal features of each of the currently most widely used systems.

HOW TO SAMPLE GASES

Gases are best measured right after they leave and just before they enter the patient, and by either a sidestream or a mainstream method. With a sidestream analyzer, gases are aspirated close to the patient's mouth (Figure 15.1) and carried to a remote analyzer. The advantage of sidestream analyzers is that the sampling tube is lightweight, inexpensive, and easy to arrange for gas sampling whether the patient is intubated or breathing spontaneously. The aspirated gas can be analyzed for different gases by different methods in the process.

The disadvantage of the sidestream analyzer is that for analysis, gas must be removed from the breathing system in amounts ranging from 50 to 200 ml/min or more. With some sidestream analyzers, the gas sampling flow can be adjusted, for example, to 50 or 150 ml/min. A lower sampling flow rate has been suggested for pediatric patients. However, a sampling flow rate less than 100 ml/min causes damping and poor resolution of the capnogram (Figure 15.2). End-tidal values are under-reported and inspiratory values are falsely elevated; the problem is aggravated at high respiratory rates, most common in children.[1] With sidestream analyzers, the aspirated gas must be disposed of, either by funneling it into a scavenging system or by returning it to the patient. Returning the gas necessitates filtering to prevent cross-contamination among patients.

Alternatively, the gas can be analyzed as it enters or leaves the patient by the mainstream, or "on-airway," method (Figure 15.3). Because it sits astride the airway, the mainstream analyzer avoids the disadvantages of the sidestream analyzer. The

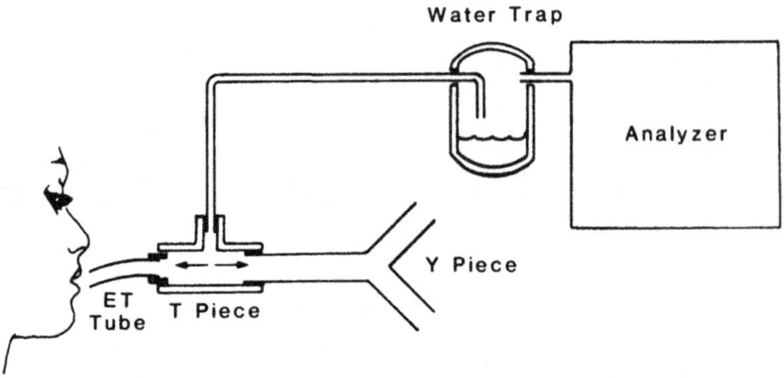

FIGURE 15.1 *In sidestream sampling, the respired gases are aspirated at a controlled flow rate from the breathing circuit, near the endotracheal (ET) tube. (Modified with permission from Gravenstein JS, Paulus DA, Hayes TJ: Capnography in clinical practice. Stoneham, MA: Butterworths, 1989:142.)*

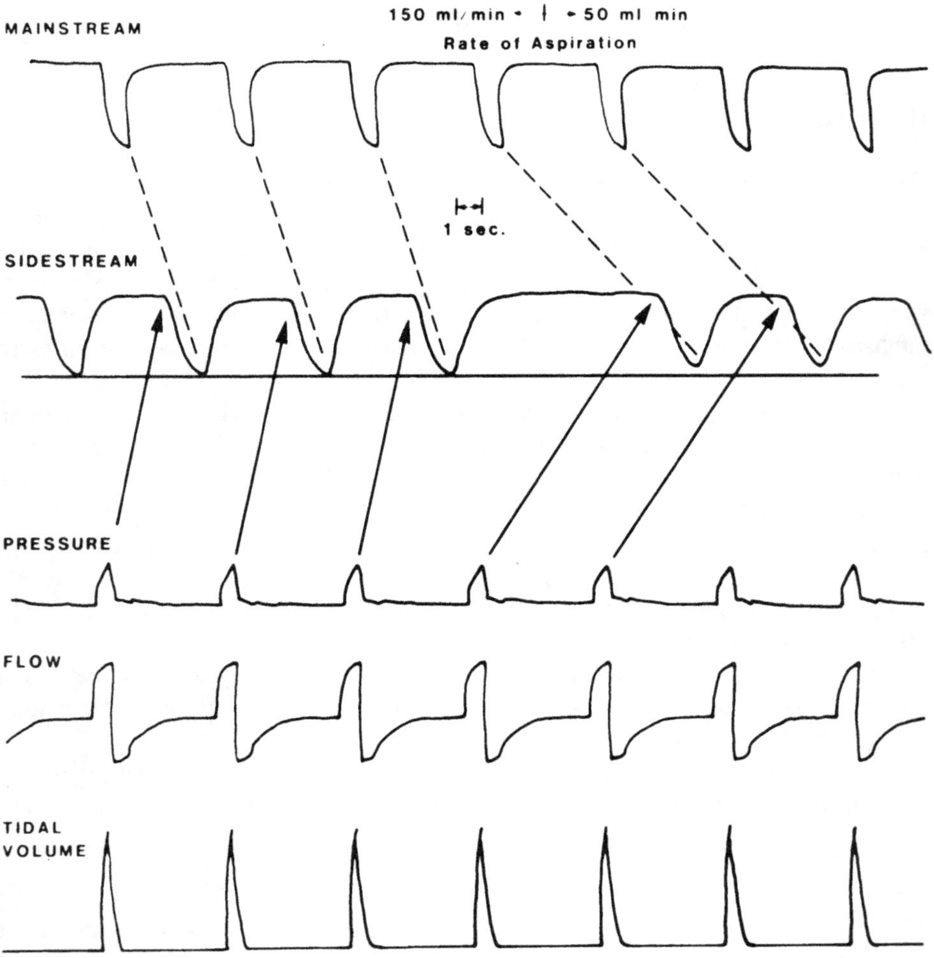

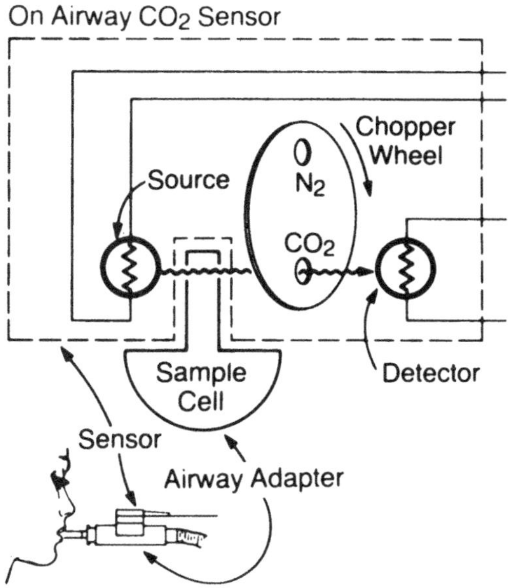

FIGURE 15.3 *A mainstream, or on-airway, sensor of a capnometer (Hewlett Packard). (Reproduced with permission from Gravenstein JS, Paulus DA, Hayes TJ: Capnography in clinical practice. Stoneham, MA: Butterworths, 1989:119.)*

disadvantage of the mainstream analyzer lies in the cuvette, which contains the analyzer and thus tends to be bulkier and heavier than the sampling connector of sidestream analyzers. The mainstream analyzer cannot combine different technologic innovations in the analysis of gases; it is enough of an accomplishment to package into a small cuvette one technologic means for analyzing one category of gas. Both sidestream and mainstream analyzers have found faithful proponents. This indicates that their advantages and disadvantages appear to be balanced.

◀ **FIGURE 15.2** *To demonstrate the effect of sampling flow rate on waveforms, carbon dioxide was infused into a mechanical lung, which was mechanically ventilated with an anesthesia machine with a circle breathing system and ventilator. Tracings are* (from top to bottom) *a capnogram from a mainstream analyzer (Hewlett Packard); a capnogram from a sidestream analyzer (Datascope), which reflects the decrease in sampling flow rate from 150 ml/min to 50 ml/min by not returning to baseline during phase I and falsely indicating rebreathing; a pressure waveform in the breathing circle; a flow waveform, the upstroke indicating inspiration; and a tidal volume waveform. The stippled lines and arrows link events to the time they were recorded by the particular waveform. (Modified with permission from Gravenstein JS, Paulus DA, Hayes TJ: Capnography in clinical practice. Stoneham, MA: Butterworths, 1989:15.)*

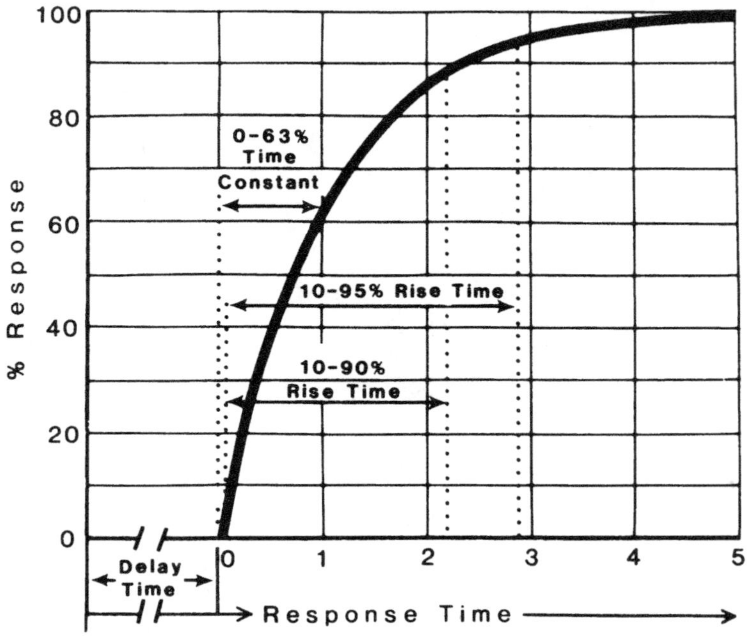

FIGURE 15.4 *The response time of a gas analyzer is the sum of the delay time (travel of gas from sampling site to analyzer) and the rise time. Rise time from 0 to 63% is also called the measurement time constant. (Modified with permission from Gravenstein JS, Paulus DA, Hayes TJ: Capnography in clinical practice. Stoneham, MA: Butterworths, 1989:102.)*

RESPONSE TIME OF GAS ANALYZERS

The time from the moment the gas sample becomes available for assay (e.g., as the gas leaves the mouth of the patient) to the moment the results of the analysis appear on the display panel of the instrument, which is the response time, can be viewed as being comprised of delay time and rise time. Delays are encountered when the gas must travel through a capillary from the patient's airway or ventilator to the analyzer. All sidestream analyzers have delay (or lag or transit) times. Low sampling flow rate of gas, large diameter of sampling capillary, long capillary, and the presence of a filter prolong the delay time.[2] Delay time for many sidestream analyzers is measured in seconds. Rise time has to do with the inherent speed with which the instrument can analyze the sample once it enters the analyzer. Typically, rise times are given for 10% to 90% of full response, usually measured in milliseconds (Figure 15.4).

THE PRESENTATION OF GAS ANALYSIS

Early capnographs relied on digital reports of $ETCO_2$. Eventually it was recognized that the task of identifying the peak end-tidal value is complex and that algorithms to accomplish this are not universally successful. For example, a sophisticated algorithm

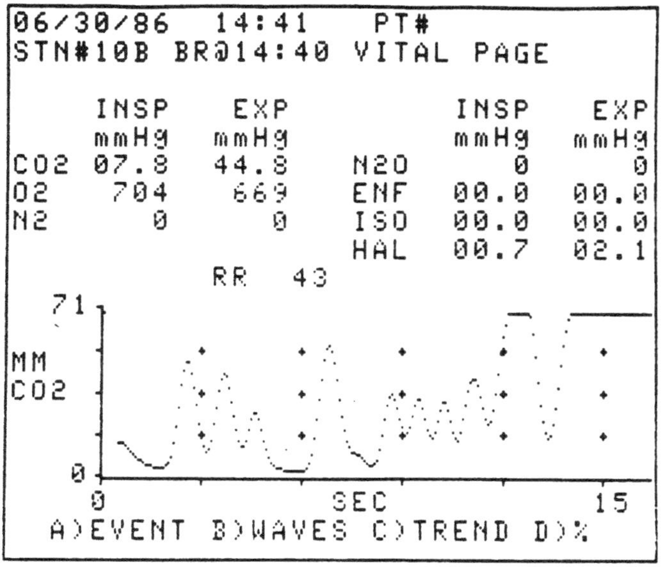

FIGURE 15.5 *Capnogram versus capnometric values. The page shown is from a mass spectrometer with a sophisticated algorithm that reported the wrong end-tidal carbon dioxide concentration in a child in respiratory distress. The digitally reported value for end-tidal (exp) carbon dioxide was 44.8 mm Hg; the true end-tidal value, however, was greater than 70 mm Hg. The error would not have been detected had the clinician not inspected the capnogram. Insp denotes inspiratory; ENF, enflurane; ISO, isoflurane; and HAL, halothane. (Modified with permission from Gravenstein JS, Paulus DA, Hayes TJ: Capnography in clinical practice. Stoneham, MA: Butterworths, 1989:6.)*

in one system gave erroneous data (Figure 15.5) at a time when inspection of the capnogram made it obvious that the digital information was not correct. Even though algorithms have been refined (Figure 15.6), no clinician should be satisfied with instruments that do not make available for inspection the actual curves tracing the changing gas concentration during several consecutive respiratory cycles.[3]

ANALYZERS THAT SUBSERVE MEASUREMENT OF ALL PHYSIOLOGIC GASES AND ANESTHETIC AGENTS

The Mass Spectrometer

As the name implies, the molecular masses of substances—here, gases and vapors—can be identified, and their concentrations measured. Toward that end, small samples of a gas are aspirated into a strong vacuum and are ionized and analyzed. To accomplish this, the magnetic-sector mass spectrometer uses a high voltage to accelerate the ions and a magnet to separate them for analysis. The quadrupole mass spectrometer employs a combined direct current and radio-frequency field to separate the ions.

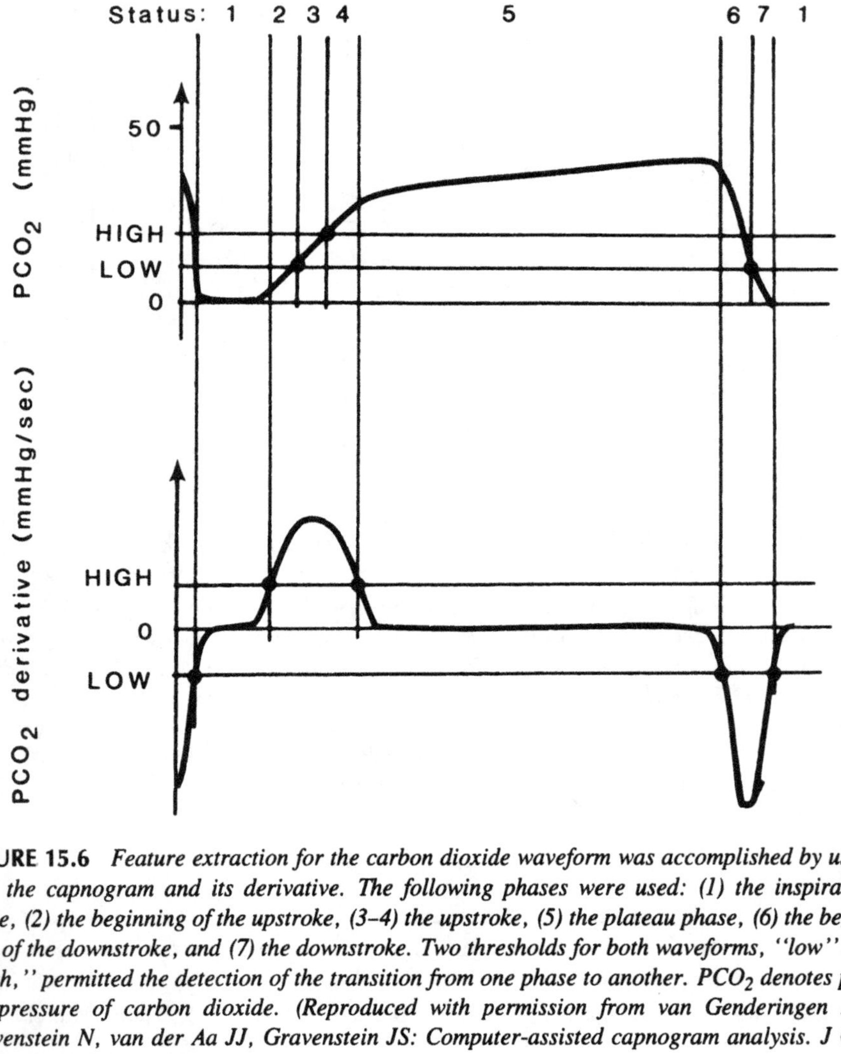

FIGURE 15.6 *Feature extraction for the carbon dioxide waveform was accomplished by using both the capnogram and its derivative. The following phases were used: (1) the inspiratory phase, (2) the beginning of the upstroke, (3–4) the upstroke, (5) the plateau phase, (6) the beginning of the downstroke, and (7) the downstroke. Two thresholds for both waveforms, "low" and "high," permitted the detection of the transition from one phase to another. PCO_2 denotes partial pressure of carbon dioxide. (Reproduced with permission from van Genderingen HR, Gravenstein N, van der Aa JJ, Gravenstein JS: Computer-assisted capnogram analysis. J Clin Monit 1987; 3:194–200.)*

Mass spectrometry is not something that can be packaged into a mainstream analyzer. Indeed, a first-generation mass spectrometer was so expensive that one had to serve up to a dozen rooms. This required sampling capillaries strung from operating rooms to a central mass spectrometer, which resulted in two delays: the gas had to travel a long way, and after an analysis of gases in room one, the patient and anesthetist in that room had to wait until the mass spectrometer had analyzed gases from all the other stations on line before the spectrometer finally could collect the next gas sample. Two-minute delays between samples were not uncommon in these systems, depending on the number of rooms being monitored and the number of breaths being analyzed in each room. To shorten the time between sampling, the multiple-room mass spectrometer can be set to collect only two breaths per room; often, that is enough. The other trick calls for a form of multiplexing.[4] Gas is sampled continuously from all stations (operating rooms) at 1.5 ml/sec and then sent to a scavenging system. When the mass spectrometer is ready to analyze gas from a station, a valve between the sampling capillary and the spectrometer opens, and gas flows at an accelerated rate under the influence of the strong vacuum of the spectrometer. The 20 sec of respiratory data stored in the 100-ft-long capillary linking the patient to the spectrometer rushes into the spectrometer and, within about 6 sec, two breaths are analyzed. The data lose some definition in the process, but the loss has been found to be acceptable.[5]

Smaller and less expensive mass spectrometers are now becoming available so that one unit can be dedicated to one operating room. Mass spectrometers can measure oxygen, carbon dioxide, nitrogen, and all anesthetic agents simultaneously and with good accuracy (whether an agent is present or absent makes no difference, as long as provisions are made for analysis of the agent). The device always makes the sum of all gases in a sample equal to 100%, taking argon (about 1% in air) into account and assuming that no unknown gas is present. This function has its bright and dark sides: bright because it automatically compensates for drift; dark because if ions appear in the analyzer that were not anticipated or for which no measurement provisions had been prepared, the results will be wrong for one of two reasons.[6–8] First, the strange gas may "tickle" one of the collection plates and cause the spectrometer to give a wrong reading. Second, when the strange ions are not detected but make up a clinically significant percentage of the gas sample, the volume occupied by the invisible gas will be attributed to identifiable gases, and the reading will be wrong. Check with the manufacturer about how a given instrument handles helium or other noble gases.

False reports by a mass spectrometer are dangerous if not recognized. Imagine that an F_{IO_2} of 0.1 is falsely reported as 0.2 and a $P_{ET}CO_2$ of 40 mm Hg is falsely reported as 70 mm Hg!

Infrared Spectroscopy

The molecules in gases are aquiver, vibrating in frequencies preordained by the masses of their atoms and the bonds that fetter them together. When exposed to energies sympathetic to these vibrations, the polyatomic molecules absorb the energies, and their vibrations intensify. To detect the molecules and gauge their abundance, we can either measure how much the energy was attenuated or record how much energy the molecules gained. Infrared spectroscopy does the former, the photoacoustic method the latter. In either case, we must select infrared wavelengths that best excite the molecules. Nitrous oxide, carbon dioxide, and carbon monoxide share a band of wavelengths (between 4 and 5 μm), which causes difficulties in separating these molecules spectroscopically. Fortunately, they respond differently, if not as strongly, to other wavelengths.

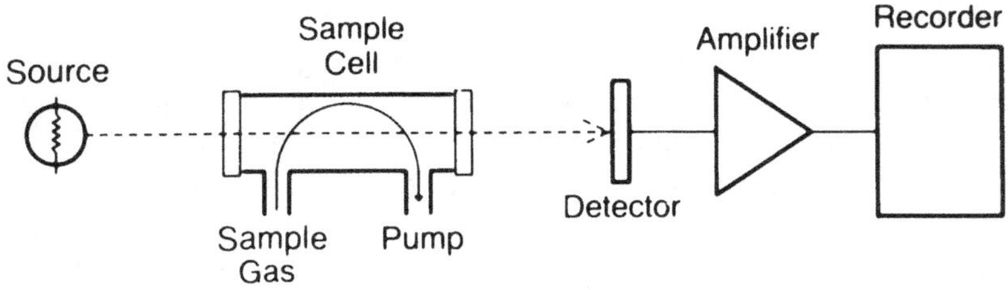

FIGURE 15.7 *An infrared single-beam capnometer. The source and detector are broad-band and nonselective. This design would work if carbon dioxide were the only absorber in the sample gas. (Reproduced with permission from Gravenstein JS, Paulus DA, Hayes TJ: Capnography in clinical practice. Stoneham, MA: Butterworths, 1989:115.)*

All infrared devices employ a source of infrared light, which shines through the gas sample. In many, a detector measures how much the light is attenuated by the gas sample (Figure 15.7). Refinements can be incorporated; for example, a second beam of infrared light can be guided through a reference cell containing a known gas for comparison; optical filters can be inserted to remove undesirable wavelengths; cells with different gases can be interposed; and mirrors can split the infrared light or collect it again. In order to generate an alternating signal that lends stability and heightens sensitivity, many devices use a chopper, a disk with holes that spins in the light path to cause darkness to cycle with light.[9]

Many infrared analyzers are not able to distinguish between different anesthetics. Instead, the user must indicate which inhalation anesthetic is in use. When the analyzer is set for one agent while a different one is administered to the patient, gross errors are possible. Guyton and Gravenstein described an analyzer that worked well when the settings were correct, but reported 6.5% anesthetic agent when 1% enflurane was present and the analyzer was incorrectly set for halothane.[10] Similar errors were observed when isoflurane was present and the analyzer was set for halothane. Conversely, when the vaporizer was set for isoflurane or enflurane but halothane was present, the analyzer grossly underreported the concentration of the agent. With the vaporizer set for either enflurane or isoflurane, insignificant errors were noted when isoflurane or enflurane, respectively, were given. Infrared analyzers when incorrectly set differ considerably in the degree to which they misrepresent gas concentrations. This limitation of the current crop of infrared analyzers is not shared by methods relying on mass spectrometry or Raman technology.

Photoacoustic Measurement

We are surrounded by physical phenomena that delight us when we discover them. One of them, first described over 100 years ago, allows us to hear music made by the sun's rays hitting the earth. Well, "music" may be overstating it, but the sun will speak to us about the concentration of gases in a sample when we arrange things just right. When we apply energy—for example, infrared light—to gas molecules capable of

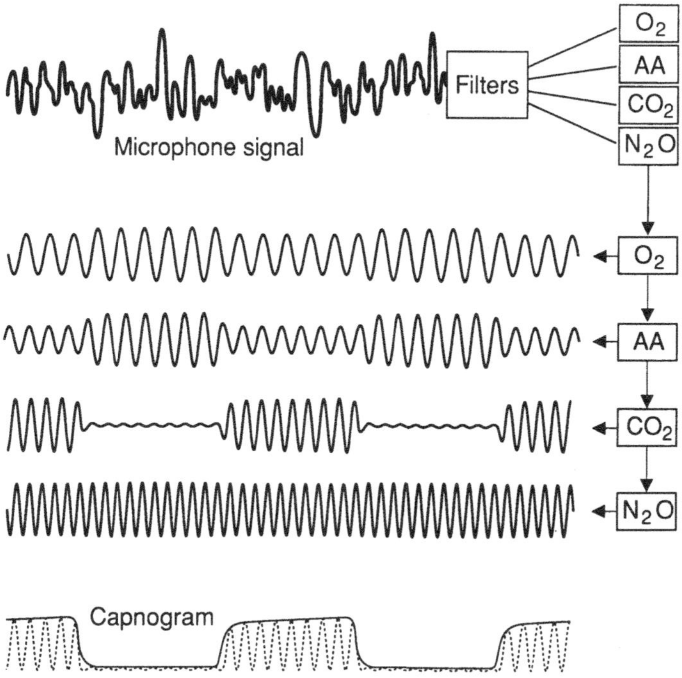

FIGURE 15.8 *The complex signal* (top trace) *received by a microphone in a photoacoustic gas analyzer, the dissected waveforms showing what each gas contributed to the complex signal, and a capnogram* (bottom trace). *AA denotes anesthetic agent. (Printed with permission from Brüel and Kjaer, Naerum, Denmark.)*

absorbing that energy, the gas will expand. As soon as the energy is withdrawn, the gas will contract to its original state. If we turn the energy (the infrared light) on and off rapidly enough, the gas in a closed chamber will expand and contract and generate pressure waves (Figure 15.8). As sound waves and pressure waves are but one expression of the same phenomenon, a microphone can be used to measure the energy absorbed by the molecules. More molecules, more absorbed energy, bigger pressure wave, more sound. Instead of turning a light on and off rapidly, a wheel with holes (a chopper wheel [Figure 15.9]) spins between light source and gas sample and, thus, permits the passage of the light beam only when another holes comes by. Carbon dioxide, nitrous oxide, and halogenated anesthetics can absorb the energy. In order to analyze several gases simultaneously in one sample, as many light filters as there are gases to be analyzed are interposed between the path of the infrared light and the sample. Each filter admits only the wavelength best absorbed by the specific agent in question. By cutting slits at different intervals in the chopper wheel and matching the slits to filters, the instrument can excite each gas in a predetermined sequence and can then record the sounds—and thus the concentrations—of different gases in the sample.

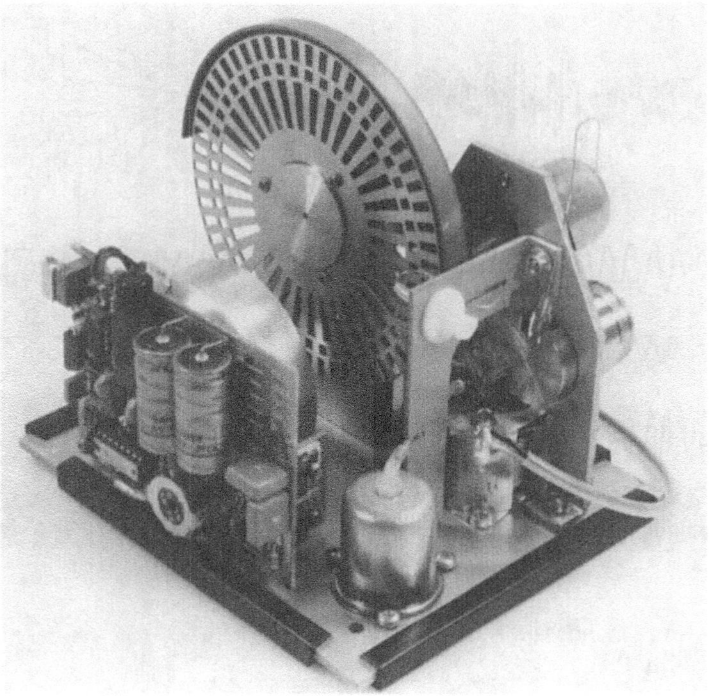

FIGURE 15.9 *The prominent chopper wheel of a medical gas analyzer (Brüel and Kjaer).*

Magnetoacoustic Analysis of Oxygen

Oxygen, that cardinal succor of life itself, maintains a special place among the gases by being strongly paramagnetic and by being consumed by some analyzers. Both qualities have been pressed into service by oxygen monitors.

Paramagnetic Oxygen Analyzer

Molecules that are repelled by magnets are called diamagnetic; those that are attracted, paramagnetic. Many substances exhibit paramagnetic properties, among them oxygen and substances with free radicals. Linus Pauling suggested that these properties of oxygen could be exploited for the analysis of oxygen. In one type of paramagnetic oxygen analyzer, the gas is attracted by a magnet and displaces glass balls filled with nitrogen in the process. The displacement is measured; the more displacement, the more oxygen.

Paramagnetic oxygen analyzers are accurate and can respond rapidly, provided that the geometry of the analyzing chamber assures quick washout of oxygen as new gas comes in for analysis. That was not the case in some of the older analyzers. Paramagnetic devices that take advantage of the capability for rapid response can be used to display the changing concentration of oxygen in respired gases.

Acoustic measurement also can exploit the paramagnetic properties of oxygen.[1] Oxygen exposed to a magnetic field that is made to oscillate will contract, expand, and thereby generate pressure waves that are proportional to the concentration of oxygen. The pressure waves are detected by microphone. Ambient air serves as a standard for comparison. Thus, the acoustic method can both detect and measure oxygen, carbon dioxide, nitrous oxide, and the halogenated anesthetics.

Polarographic Oxygen Analyzer

Oxygen reacting with metal and water is reduced to hydroxyl ions. The process generates a current that can be measured and made to correspond to the concentration of oxygen overlying the electrode. The electrode itself consists of a cathode made of platinum, gold, or silver (not only to pay homage to the queen of life-sustaining gases but also to prevent or delay oxidation of the metal) under a layer of electrolyte solution covered by a membrane poorly permeable to oxygen. A current applied to the metal sets the stage for the reduction of oxygen. This consumption causes no difficulty in oxygen analyzers of gas (rather than blood), as enough oxygen flows by to replenish what has been used up. Because heat accelerates the diffusion of oxygen through the membrane, the temperature must be monitored by the instrument and the results corrected for warming or cooling of the electrode.

Polarographic analyzers function well, are inexpensive, and come armed with alarms for low or high readings, but they are abominably slow to respond to changes in oxygen concentration. Their response time must be reckoned in seconds, sometimes dozens of them, rather than milliseconds. Therefore, polarographic oxygen analyzers in the inspiratory hose can serve as safety monitors—is a sufficient concentration of oxygen being given and is it really oxygen that comes out of the fresh gas supply?—but cannot show differences between inspired and end-tidal concentrations of oxygen. The position of these analyzers in the inspiratory hose of circle systems has the advantage that the gas tends to be dry; some polarographic analyzers are sensitive to moisture. The response time of polarographic oxygen analyzers has improved over the years through both better design and the use of clever software.

The Fuel Cell, or Self-Polarizing Electrode

Instead of applying a current to the metal, a metal for the reference electrode can be selected that is sufficiently electronegative to drive the reaction with oxygen. The principles involved for these battery-free electrodes are the same as described above for the polarographic electrode. They are no faster than the battery-driven polarographic electrodes. Instruments with no alarm capability do not meet the minimal monitoring standards of the ASA.

RAMAN SCATTERING

Dust dancing in sunlight gives evidence that light can be scattered by matter. When the light not only is scattered but also suffers a change in wavelength as it hits and excites molecules, we speak of Raman scattering. The wavelengths that emerge after the collision of light with polyatomic molecules are marked by the nature of the molecules with which they collided, and by their abundance. Thus, Raman scattering can be used in the analysis of respiratory gases.[11] Because Raman scattering can be employed to analyze many different polyatomic gases simultaneously, it can trace the changing concentrations of oxygen, nitrogen, carbon dioxide, and anesthetic agents and can do so rapidly enough to generate graphs.[12,13] Multi-gas monitors using a laser for a light source and exploiting the Raman phenomenon are now available for clinical use.

REFERENCES

1. Gravenstein N, McLaughlin G. van Genderingen HR, Lampotang S: Effect of respiratory rate, tidal volume, and sample volume on pediatric capnography. Anesthesiology 1985; 63:A182 (abstr)
2. Frei FJ, Zbinden AM, Weckler H, Thomson D: Parameters influencing the response time of volatile anesthetic monitors. Int J Clin Monit Comput 1989; 6:21–30
3. van Genderingen HR, Gravenstein N, van der Aa JJ, Gravenstein JS: Computer-assisted capnogram analysis. J Clin Monit 1987; 3:194–200
4. Ozanne GM, Young WG, Mazzei WJ, Severinghaus JW: Multipatient anesthetic mass spectrometry: Rapid analysis of data stored in long catheters. Anesthesiology 1981; 55: 62–67
5. Severinghaus JW: Monitoring anesthetic and respiratory gases. In: Blitt CD, ed. Monitoring in anesthesia and critical care medicine. New York: Churchill Livingstone, 1985: 265–290
6. Gravenstein JS, Gravenstein N, van der Aa JJ, et al: Pitfalls with mass spectrometry in clinical anesthesia. Int J Clin Monit Comp 1984; 1:27–34
7. Gravenstein N, Theisen GJ, Knudsen AK: Misleading mass spectrometry reading caused by an aerosol propellant. Anesthesiology 1985; 62:70–72
8. Siegel M, Gravenstein N: Evaluation of helium interference with mass spectrometry. Anesth Analg 1988; 67:887–889
9. Gravenstein JS, Paulus DA, Hayes TJ: Capnography in clinical practice. Stoneham, MA: Butterworths, 1989: 114–121
10. Guyton DC, Gravenstein N: Infrared analysis of volatile anesthetics: Impact of monitor agent setting, volatile mixtures, and alcohol. J Clin Monit, in press
11. West GA, Barrett JJ, Siebert DR, Reddy KV: Photoacoustic spectroscopy. Rev Sci Instrum 1983; 54:797–817
12. Westenskow DR, Coleman DL: Can the Raman scattering analyzer compete with mass spectrometers: An affirmative reply. J Clin Mon 1989; 5:34–36
13. Westenskow DR, Smith KW, Coleman DL, Gregonis DE, Van Wagenen RA: Clinical evaluation of a Raman scattering multiple gas analyzer for the operating room. Anesthesiology 1988; 70:350–355

Chapter 16

About Hemoglobin Saturation Measurements

Much direct and indirect evidence points to hypoxemia as the most common final event in anesthetic disaster that leads to permanent brain injury and death. Hypoxemia reduces hemoglobin saturation, which leads to cyanosis. Unfortunately, cyanosis is not only a late sign of significant desaturation, but its detection depends on skin pigmentation and perfusion and on the hemoglobin concentration in blood. In some patients who become cold, cyanosis of the lips and fingertips develops; a little rubbing of the tissue will bring arterial blood into the underperfused tissue, and the cyanosis will disappear. Anemic patients may be quite hypoxemic yet their blood may show no evidence of cyanosis. Cyanosis is not a reliable clinical sign of hypoxemia.[1]

When pulse oximetry provided a noninvasive method for monitoring the saturation of oxygen in arterial blood, anesthetists embraced the technology enthusiastically. I cannot recall a monitoring method that has gained general acceptance as rapidly and as widely as pulse oximetry has. As of 1990, this monitoring modality joins the list of requisite monitors enumerated in the Standards for Basic Intra-operative Monitoring published by the American Society of Anesthesiologists.

The method is simple to apply, but the user must understand its principles of operation in order to appreciate its power and its limitations.

METHODOLOGY OF PULSE OXIMETRY

Color appears when some of the light shining on or through a substance is absorbed. When hemoglobin picks up oxygen in the lungs, it changes from dusky bluish-red to bright red. Measuring the color of blood, therefore, makes it possible to estimate how much of the hemoglobin in the blood is bluish and reduced, and how much is red and oxygenated. The light absorbed (or extinguished) by hemoglobin extends from red (wavelengths between 650 nm and 750 nm) to the infrared (900 nm to 1000 nm) region. Extinction curves for oxyhemoglobin (HbO_2), carboxyhemoglobin (HbCO), reduced hemoglobin (Hb), and methemoglobin (HbMET) show why HbO_2 and HbCO impart a redder color to blood than do Hb and HbMET (Figure 16.1).

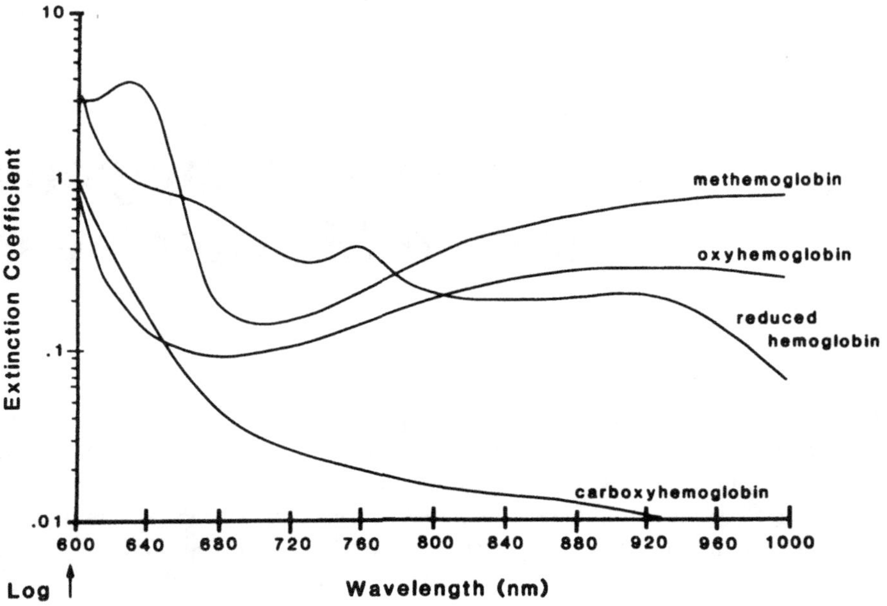

FIGURE 16.1 *Hemoglobin extinction curves, showing relationship of reduced hemoglobin, oxyhemoglobin, carboxyhemoglobin, and methemoglobin to light absorption. (Courtesy of Ohmeda, Denver, Colorado.)*

The tissue of a finger or earlobe extinguishes much more light than does hemoglobin because there is so much more tissue than blood. A brilliant solution was necessary to identify the light absorbed by Hb and distinguish it from the much larger absorption by tissue: enter pulse oximetry. If we shine a light through a finger or an earlobe, the light emerging on the other side waxes and wanes in intensity with the pulsation of blood because the tissue swells a little with every heartbeat. A plethysmogram can record these volume changes over time. Light absorption by live tissue can be divided into two components, pulsatile and nonpulsatile (Figure 16.2). The pulsatile component arises almost exclusively from the pulsation of arteries and arterioles, the nonpulsatile from tissue, bones, skin, and the nonpulsatile component of arterial and venous blood. Therefore, subtracting the nonpulsatile signal from the total signal yields the signals of pulsating arterial blood. Thank you, Mr. Takuo Aoyaki, for describing this and pointing the way to pulse oximetry.[2]

Several engineering feats have to be accomplished in order to extract from this signal the information about the ratio of Hbo_2 to Hb.[3-5] For one, the light extinction of the two wavelengths, typically 660 nm and 940 nm, is measured repeatedly during one heartbeat. As the tissue swells during systole, light extinction also increases. From a range of values gathered many times during each heartbeat, the instrument must calculate a reasonable single estimate most representative of the percentage of Hbo_2. To accomplish this, it is necessary to present a weighted average for several heartbeats or

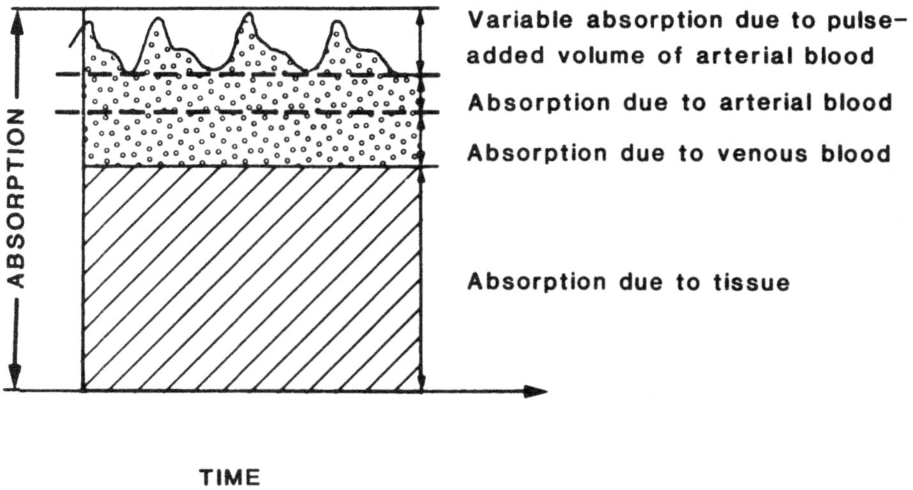

FIGURE 16.2 *Tissue composite, showing dynamic and static components affecting light absorption. (Courtesy of Ohmeda.)*

several seconds (usually 2 to 10). While the extinction varies with each heartbeat, the strength of the pulsations also varies with changes in arterial pressure and vascular tone. Therefore, the instrument must adjust either the amplification of the signal, the strength of the light, or both in response to such changes. This has led many manufacturers to adjust the intensity of the light automatically so as to assure an even response, regardless of fluctuations in the plethysmogram owing to the fluctuation of the thickness of the finger or the ear over several heartbeats. This variability can be turned to an advantage by using the variability of the plethysmogram to estimate volume status.[6] The height of the waveform varies with mechanical ventilation more in hypovolemic than in normovolemic patients (Figure 16.3). An instrument in which the user can adjust and fix the gain factor of the pulse oximeter permits the observation of waveform variability. With automatic adjustment of the gain, this is more difficult or impossible.

A number of disturbances complicate matters for the instrument. Ambient light, movement, and electronic artifact cause troublesome interferences that must be filtered out as best as possible. Some fluorescent lights, for example, emit in the 660-nm region, which can substantially distort analysis by a pulse oximeter.[7]

Finally, the instrument must be calibrated—and that is no easy matter. Direct comparisons for calibration are not available; the manufacturers use algorithms based on in vitro measurements and clinical studies. The accuracy of the instruments varies greatly and is generally better for values above 80% saturation and worse for values lower than that.[8-10] While this diminishes the value of pulse oximetry and demonstrates its limitation as a scientific instrument, it does not negate the clinical value of pulse oximetry when patients are slipping into hypoxia. The message "low oxygen sat-

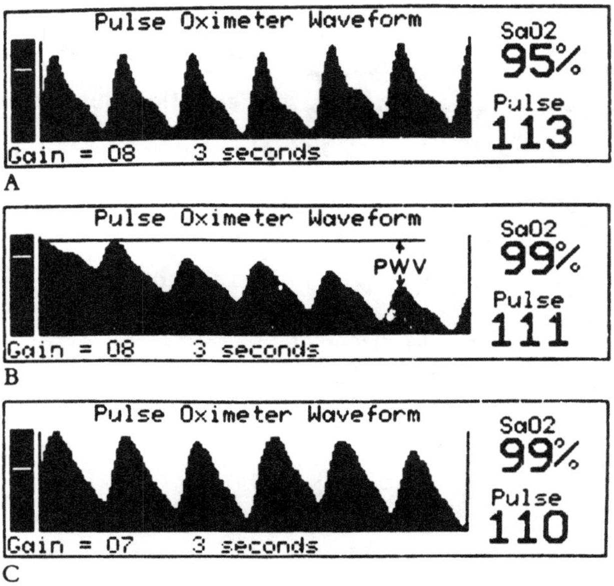

FIGURE 16.3 *Pulse oximeter waveform representation. When the patient arrived in the operating room* (A), *central venous pressure (CVP) was 8 mm Hg. Little variation was seen in the waveform with positive pressure ventilation. After third space and blood loss* (B), *CVP was 4 to 5 mm Hg. The pulse waveform varied with respiration. The method for measuring pulse waveform variation (PWV) is shown. After fluid resuscitation* (C), *CVP was 8 mm Hg. The pulse waveform no longer shows significant variation with respiration. (Reproduced with permission from Partridge BL: Use of pulse oximetry as a noninvasive indicator of intravascular volume status. J Clin Monit 1987; 3:263–268.)*

uration'' carries great meaning for the clinician, even if the exact level of hypoxemia cannot be ascertained. Significant disparities exist among pulse oximeters from different manufacturers, and often between data from probes applied to the finger and ear lobe.[10] The circumstances under which hypoxia began can also contribute to the differences; for example, when hypoxia accompanies hyperventilation, finger blood flow may be affected differently from when hypoxia has existed for some time and ventilation is not affected.[10]

WHAT THE PULSE OXIMETER READS

We now have to come back to the problem of how HbMET and HbCO can generate difficulties for oximetry (Figure 16.1). The absorption of light by these two moieties of Hb contribute to that of HbO_2 (particularly HbCO) and Hb (particularly HbMET). Fortunately, the concentrations of these two forms of Hb are normally so low that they can be ignored. HbMET level usually lies below 3% of total Hb. Elevated levels are seen in patients with idiopathic methemoglobinemia, after the ingestion of drugs (e.g., phenacetin or nitroglycerin) that can overwhelm the reducing mechanism of the red cell, or after the inhalation or ingestion of butyl or isobutyl nitrites.[11] Even a modest elevation to less than 5 g/dL of methemoglobinemia results in cyanosis, though the patient may be asymptomatic. With a higher level, the patient suffers the consequences of hypoxemia, as the HbMET carries no oxygen. Pulse oximetry becomes unreliable at higher HbMET. In an animal experiment, pulse oximeters tended to overestimate the true saturation of Hb in the presence of HbMET.[12] Troublesome is the observation in this study that decreasing saturation of Hb in the presence of HbMET was not reflected by the pulse oximeter.

Rarer than HbMET is sulfhemoglobin (HbSULF), in which sulfur in the porphyrin ring gives the Hb a blue-green hue.[13] It too causes cyanosis and is an indolent transporter of oxygen.

In nonsmokers (who do not work in tunnels traversed by automobiles that spew forth carbon monoxide and who are not otherwise exposed to carbon monoxide), HbCO in blood is less than 2% of total Hb. Up to 10% of total Hb in heavy smokers might be occupied by carbon monoxide. HbCO can reach 50% or more in patients poisoned with carbon monoxide after inhaling smoke or the exhaust fumes of gasoline engines. Here, pulse oximetry cannot be used to assess the saturation of Hb with oxygen. A patient with 10% HbCO and 90% O_2Hb may appear to have a hemoglobin saturation of 97% or 98% according to a pulse oximeter, when true O_2Hb must in fact be 90% or less.[3] Fetal hemoglobin[14] and bilirubin[15] appear to cause no difficulties for the pulse oximeter.

EXTERNAL DYES THAT AFFECT PULSE OXIMETRY

If naturally occurring substances can confound the pulse oximeter, so can dyes that are injected intravenously. Worst, perhaps, is methylene blue. The greater its concentration in blood, the lower an oxygen saturation—down to 65%—will the pulse oximeter report. Methylene blue (2 to 5 mg/kg) lowered pulse oximetry readings for 10 min to 60 min and indocyanine green (0.5 to 2.0 mg/kg) for 1 min to 15 min.[16] Indocyanine green distorts the data less and indigo carmine, least.[17,18] Fluorescein is without effect. Some nail polish affects the accuracy of pulse oximetry; because one cannot predict which will interfere with the instrument, all nail polish should be removed.

REPORTING OXYGEN SATURATION

Ideally, when speaking of percent hemoglobin saturation, we would like to report the ratio of saturated hemoglobin (HbO_2) to total Hb (including HbO_2, Hb, HbMET, HbCO, and HbSULF) times 100. This has been called the *fractional* saturation of hemoglobin, or fractional SaO_2, where "a" signifies arterial. As we have seen, pulse oximetry cannot assess HbMET, HbCO, or HbSULF. In recognizing that limitation, we speak of a percentage of *functional* saturation of hemoglobin and understand that this

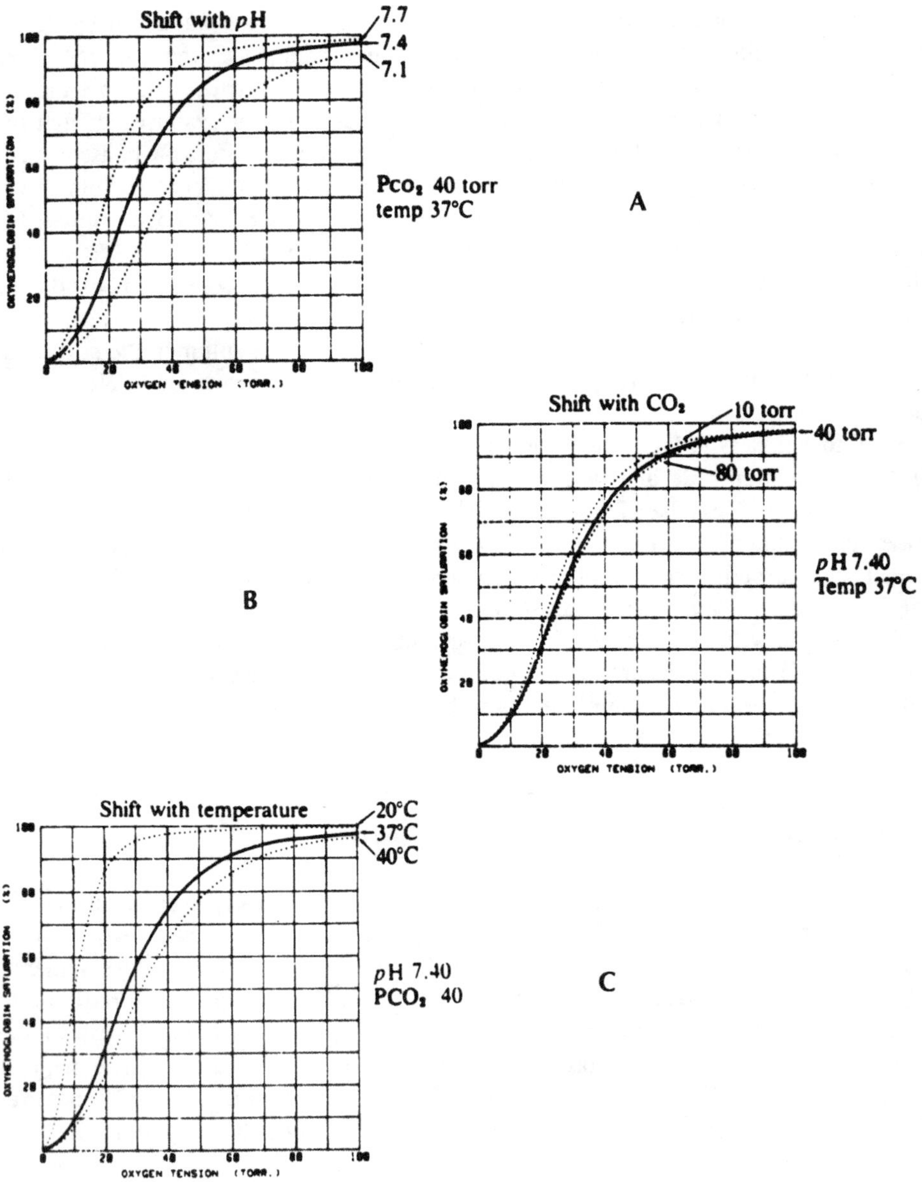

FIGURE 16.4 *Saturation of hemoglobin with oxygen. The typical S-shaped dissociation curve can be shifted to the left (with loss of H^+ ions, decrease of temperature, reduction of 2,3-diphosphoglycerate) and to the right (with gain of H^+ ions; rise of temperature, increase of 2,3-diphosphoglycerate). Observe that carbon dioxide affects the position of the curve only a little, provided that the pH is constant. Usually, pH shifts with changes in carbon dioxide tension (PCO_2) and, thus, the dissociation curve also shifts. Only the effects of pH* (A), *PCO_2* (B), *and temperature* (C) *are shown, because these are purposefully manipulated during anesthesia; however, 2,3-diphosphoglycerate is not. (Reproduced with permission from Gravenstein JS, Paulus DA: Clinical monitoring practice, 2nd ed. Philadelphia: J.B. Lippincott, 1987:162.)*

refers to 100 times the quotient of $Hbo_2/(Hbo_2 + Hb)$, which is approximately what pulse oximetry measures. But, as there are several variables over which we have little influence, the convention now widely adopted calls the oxygen saturation measured by pulse oximetry SpO_2, where *p* signifies pulse oximetry. This sets it apart from SaO_2, which is reserved for the saturation of arterial blood as measured in the blood with a cooximeter or as calculated from PaO_2, corrected for temperature and pH.

COMPARISON OF MEASUREMENTS BY PULSE OXIMETRY AND BLOOD GAS ANALYSIS

The oft-depicted sigmoid relationship between oxygen saturation and hemoglobin (Figure 16.4) reminds us that under normal circumstances the pulse oximeter will report 100% saturation, whether the PaO_2 is 150 mm Hg, 300 mm Hg, or 600 mm Hg or is hyperbaric at 1200 mm Hg. But on the lower scale, oxygen saturation will drop from 75% to 60% when the PaO_2 slides from only 40 mm Hg to 30 mm Hg. An easy rule of thumb approximates 90% SpO_2 as PaO_2 of 60 mm Hg and 30% SpO_2 as PaO_2 of 30 mm Hg. The almost linear relationship between SpO_2 and PaO_2 in this region of the dissociation diagram shows why this is so. Theoretically, therefore, pulse oximetry is more sensitive at the time of greatest concern to us—when a patient has substantial hypoxemia. Unfortunately, pulse oximeters tend to perform more accurately in the range between 80% and 100% saturation than in the lower ranges. It is important to position the pulse oximetry probe so that its light shines through the tissue covered by the skin as well as the skin in order to avoid the penumbra effect.[19] This effect leads to falsely low SpO_2 readings.

We find that the saturation values of most of our patients range between 80% and 100% saturation. Oxygen saturation is affected by changes in acid-base balance, 2,3-diphosphoglycerate, and temperature. On the surface, then, it appears that PaO_2 provides a far better measure of oxygenation than can pulse oximetry. That the latter method has won the hearts of clinicians can be attributed to several advantages of pulse oximetry over measurements of oxygen tension: pulse oximetry reports saturation almost heartbeat by heartbeat and does so noninvasively, reports heart rate along with saturation, and can generate a plethysmogram that gives information on the perfusion of the tissue. Also, besides being noninvasive, the probes are easy to apply. For these reasons, transcutaneous measurement of the partial pressure of oxygen has not been as successful as pulse oximetry (Table 16.1).[20] We still need to obtain PaO_2 clinically when we wish to calculate shunts or when we worry about patients poisoned with carbon monoxide or affected by dyes. But for moment-to-moment monitoring of oxygen saturation, pulse oximetry has established itself as an indispensable aid to the clinician in the operating room, recovery room, and intensive care unit.

Table 16.1 Comparison of Pulse Oximeter and Cutaneous Oxygen Tension Monitor

Pulse Oximeter	*Cutaneous Oxygen Tension Monitor*
Advantages	
Continuous arterial oxygen saturation	Continuous oxygen tension
No warm-up	Low cutaneous blood flow detection (indirect)
Multiple site choices	
Noninvasive	Noninvasive
No tissue injury	
Direct reading of signal strength	
No calibration	
Easy sensor application	
Heart rate gives indication of signal quality	
Disadvantages	
Ambient light can affect	Low cutaneous blood flow mars correlation with arterial O_2
No trend of PaO_2 until low (70 torr)	
Calibration not available	Warm-up required
Electrocautery causes errors	Burns skin
Motion artifact	Requires membrane changes
Pulsatile signal needed	Requires calibration
May fail with anemia	Requires site changes
Dyes may affect	Sensor application not easy
Need nonpulsatile venous pressure	No signal strength indication

Source: Barker SJ, Tremper KK: Transcutaneous oxygen tension: Physiologic variables for monitoring oxygenation. J Clin Monit 1985; 1:130–134. With permission of the author and Little, Brown Co.

REFERENCES

1. Comroe JH Jr, Botelho S: The reliability of cyanosis in the recognition of arterial anoxemia. Am J Med Sci 1947; 214:1–6
2. Severinghaus JW, Astrup PB: History of blood gas analysis. Int Anesthesiol Clin 1987; 25:167–214
3. Wukitsch MW, Petterson MT, Tobler DR, Pologe JA: Pulse oximetry: Analysis of theory, technology, and practice. J Clin Monit 1988; 4:290–301
4. Tremper KK, Barker SJ: Pulse oximetry. Anesthesiology 1989; 70:98–108
5. Alexander CM, Teller LE, Gross JB: Principles of pulse oximetry: Theoretical and practical considerations. Anesth Analg 1989; 68:368–376
6. Partridge BL: Use of pulse oximetry as a noninvasive indicator of intravascular volume status. J Clin Monit 1987; 3:263–268
7. Amar D, Neidzwski J, Wald A, Finck DA: Fluorescent light interferes with pulse oximetry. J Clin Monit 1989; 5:135–136
8. Severinghaus JW, Naifeh KH: Accuracy of response of six pulse oximeters to profound hypoxia. Anesthesiology 1987; 67:551–558
9. Nickerson BG, Sakrison C, Tremper KK: Bias and precision of pulse oximeters and arterial oximeters. Chest 1988; 93:515–517

10. Severinghaus JW, Naifeh KH, Koh SO: Errors in 14 pulse oximeters during profound hypoxia. J Clin Monit 1989; 5:72–81
11. Jaff ER: Methemoglobinemia in the differential diagnosis of cyanosis. Hosp Pract 1985; 20:92
12. Barker SJ, Tremper KK, Hyatt J: Effects of methemoglobinemia on pulse oximetry and mixed venous oximetry. Anesthesiology 1989; 70:112–117
13. Park CM, Nagel RL: Sulfhemoglobinemia: Clinical and molecular aspects. N Engl J Med 1984; 310:1597
14. Pologe JA, Raley DM: Effects of fetal hemoglobin on pulse oximetry. J Perinatol 1987; 7:324–326
15. Veyckemans F, Baele P, Guillaume JE, Willems E, Robert A, Clebaux T: Hyperbilirubinemia does not interfere with hemoglobin saturation measured by pulse oximetry. Anesthesiology 1989; 70:118–122
16. Sidi A, Paulus DA, Rush W, Gravenstein N, Davis RF: Methylene blue and indocyanine green artificially lower pulse oximetry readings of oxygen saturation: Studies in dogs. J Clin Monit 1987; 3:249–256
17. Scheller MS, Unger RJ, Kelner MJ: Effects of intravenously administered dyes on pulse oximetry reading. Anesthesiology 1986; 65:550–552
18. Sidi A, Rush WR, Paulus DA, Gravenstein N, Davis RF: Effect of fluorescein, indocyanine green, and methylene blue on the measurement of oxygen saturation by pulse oximetry. Anesthesiology 1986; 65:A132 (abstr)
19. Kelleher JF, Ruff RH: The "penumbra effect": Pulse oximeter artifact due to probe malposition is attenuated by vasoconstriction. Anesthesiology 1989; 71:A372 (abstr)
20. Barker SJ, Tremper KK, Gamel DM: A clinical comparison of transcutaneous PO_2 and pulse oximetry in the operating room. Anesth Analg 1986; 65:805–808

Index

Printed in France by Amazon
Brétigny-sur-Orge, FR

51786461R00092